# *Dancing*
# Without Danger

# *Dancing* Without Danger

### THE PREVENTION AND TREATMENT OF BALLET DANCING INJURIES

by Donald F. Featherstone

Written in collaboration with

RONA ALLEN

SOUTH BRUNSWICK AND NEW YORK: A. S. BARNES AND COMPANY

A. S. Barnes and Co., Inc.
Cranbury, New Jersey 08512

Second Printing, 1977

SBN: 498 06995 8
Printed in the United States of America

# Contents

# Foreword

The following letter was printed in "Dancing Times" in February, 1963.

## TEACHING DANGERS

Dear Sir,

I have recently been teaching the Royal Academy of Dancing's Ballet in Education syllabus to English and German pupils in Paderborn.

Their former teacher, a German, had been giving the smallest children acrobatic exercises and had forced pupils with excessive limbering exercises.

As a result of this, one child had been in hospital with a displaced hip, weakened by over-forcing the turn-out, and has to have pins to secure the hip joint. She has been like this for some months.

I think your readers may be interested and horrified to know what harm bad teaching (particularly in children's work) can do, quite apart from the danger of too early pointe work—a danger which is now, fortunately, well known.

Yours faithfully,

Nirissa Windham.

B.F.P.O. 16, Germany

It is with the aim of preventing such unfortunate incidents that this book has been written.

# Preface

Throughout the conception and writing of this book, I have been conscious that many people may doubt the wisdom of discussing the treatment of dancing injuries with teachers and parents who lack medical qualifications. Nevertheless, whether or not a teacher or parent has any such knowledge, at some time or other, she will inevitably come into contact with an injury sustained while dancing. It would appear to be preferable that she have a basic knowledge or source of information concerning these injuries, even if it only serves to alert her to her limitations in this field.

When an injury occurs, the best that a teacher can do is to try to alleviate the immediate pain and control the early symptoms. If she does this, then she is likely to lessen the length and severity of the disability period. The advice contained in this book should not tempt the teacher to assume the mantle of the physiotherapist and convert part of her studio into a clinic!

Consider the legal aspects of pupils sustaining injury on studio premises and the assessing of responsibility for negligence or faulty handling of that injury. Reading a book such as this and so acquainting herself with the rudiments of injury treatment and prevention reflects favorably upon the teacher. She is shown to have taken a positive action that could materially assist her pupils in a moment of physical stress.

I would like to thank the dancer who posed for the photographs in the book—Miss Jill Rackley, pupil of the Julie Watts School of Dancing in Southampton. But, most of all, my gratitude goes out to Rona Allen, teacher at the same school, for her unremitting technical advice and criticism during the writing of this book. The author has considerable experience with injuries sustained by players of most branches of sport, but lacks the technical background and experience necessary to fully comprehend the stresses and strains endured by the ballet dancer —surely the most artistic of all athletes? Without Rona Allen's patient and competent assistance, the book would never have got into "first position!"
*DONALD F. FEATHERSTONE*
Southampton

# Introduction

The very nature of what they are doing exposes ballet dancers to injury and strain, a situation aggravated by the unnatural or unphysiological postures that form an integral part of the art. It is an arduous, strenuous occupation, often demanding almost maximum physical output from the body. This means that any imperfection in technique or posture will inevitably result in eventual injury. A further complication arises because dancers are sometimes young and have not reached physical maturity; they are constitutionally and often psychologically incapable of sustained physical effort. Factors have to be considered which are frequently beyond the dancer's personal control—a lift in a Pas De Deux may be mistimed or the music tempo may force them to move faster or slower than they choose.

A ballet dancer is an artistic athlete. There is much that occurs on a sportsfield that can provide inspiration for the choreographer—indeed it has done so. Similarly, there are few athletes who would not benefit from the rhythm and mobility of the dancer. An athlete is said to have "style"—a quality derived from a poise attained by adjustment of the body to the athletic activity. This "style" is not merely a matter of gracefulness and charm; it is a quality, a poise of optimum adjustment—it is the most important factor in athletic success. Nearly all athletic deficiencies of a physical nature originate from some maladjustment that causes the momentum of the body to interfere with movement of the limbs. It can be fairly claimed that the principal physical deficiencies of athletes are precisely the factors in which the dancer excels.

Accepting that a dancer is an athlete, we must also accept that injury is the occupational hazard of athletics. Taken further, this indicates that a dancer, when injured, shall receive the same brisk type of treatment that returns an athlete to his sport. But now we come to the remarkable fact that in a country where games are such an essential part of national life, the subject of sports injuries has received relatively little attention. Their treatment, at any rate in the vital early stages, has been very largely empirical and often almost primitive. When one considers the frequency of injuries incurred at sport, and while dancing, it is clear that these sprains and strains do not receive a commensurable degree of attention or foresight from those responsible for their treatment. And yet their significance, not only from the athletic, but also the economic point of view, is of the greatest importance.

When we consider the dancer, particularly the professional, we see a man or woman who has a more-than-usual consciousness of his body and his physical fitness. Couple with this an environmental inclination to be artistically temperamental and we discover the existence of a mental state of anxiety and tension. For this to affect the dancer's performance, it is not even necessary to be suffering from an injury that prevents actual dancing. Many dancers, particularly those in the Corps de Ballet, with first aid, will grit their teeth and carry on in spite of the discomfort; a principal dancer will often have to drop out of a role.

However much we admire and respect the dancer who carries on while suffering pain and restriction, the fact has to be faced that the dancer must have a full range of move in every joint; if this is prevented then her ability to adequately perform is impaired. "Nursing" a painful limb or joint throws additional strain on other limbs, joints or muscles, eventually causing further injury. Thus, neglect of the "primary" condition superimposes upon it a "secondary" condition, sometimes more severe than the original injury!

On the other hand, when it is decided that complete rest is the quickest road to recovery, other considerations have to be faced. There is the psychological factor of worry, impatience and restlessness; more than that, there is the rapid diminishment of stamina and general muscle tone. In the latter connection, it has always been the policy of the author to continue exercising the uninjured parts of the body during the disability period. Known as "treat and train" it is a method that endeavors to have the injured athlete ready for full action as soon as the injury clears up.

By careful planning and adequate supervision it is possile to prevent a large percentage of injuries. Today, when a dancer is injured she has three alternatives:

1. She can visit her G. P. who usually prescribes "rest"—obviously not very attractive to the energetic and enthusiastic dancer.
   This is a sincere attempt by a recognized member of the medical profession to treat an injury. It usually fails because in these busy days the doctor

concerned has neither the time nor interest to spare on the comparatively minor troubles of an otherwise fit young person.

2. She may allow the teacher to do her best, but the teacher works only with the sparse knowledge she has acquired through sustaining the same injuries during her own dancing career. It is anticipated that this book will improve such a situation.

3. Or the dancer can treat herself, until such time as nature provides a cure or she is hobbling around with a serious chronic condition caused by neglect or incorrect treatment. This, the third alternative is, at best, a risky procedure for the young dancer.

It is the teachers and parents who can do much to alter this picture of indifference and neglect—by gaining a simple working knowledge of the more common injuries so that they can recognize them and institute elementary treatments. Conversely, they will also learn enough to know when an injury is beyond their scope and needs to be put into more qualified hands. A basic knowledge of anatomy and of physiology, together with practical experience in simple first aid, will enable the layman to accomplish a great deal for young pupils. It will also instill a sense of confidence into the dancers themselves and go a long way toward convincing their parents that their children are in good hands.

# PART I
# THE HUMAN BODY

# The Structure and Working
# of the Body

An eminent authority in the world of ballet dancing has written: *"Projection,* the currently fashionable word to describe the impact of world famous dancers, stems solely from a knowledge of the muscles of the body," Andrew Hardie ("Dancing Times," July, 1963). It is a statement backed by knowledge and experience, reflecting a consciousness of the physical strength and coordination that is required to achieve the essential grace and mastery possessed by all great dancers. Misjudgement or lack of coordination can cause loss of control leading to injury. Such eventualities can often be prevented by knowing the ranges in which a muscle can work, how a joint operates and the functioning of the various systems of the human body. It is highly desirable for a dancer, and her teachers, to have an elementary knowledge of anatomy and physiology to avert such dangers.

Anatomy is the science of bodily structure and physiology is the science of the normal function of living things; studied together they give a picture of the build-up of the human frame and the effects of exercise upon it. Every effort has been made to keep these necessary details as simple as possible within this volume, while not omitting any vital or important details.

## The Skeleton

The human body is built around, or molded upon, a bony skeleton which serves to give shape and firmness to the body, and to afford attachment for muscles which need a rigid framework in order to move body parts. Lastly, the skeleton protects important organs, such as the skull containing the brain, the chest containing the heart and lungs, and the abdomen, which has within it the stomach and intestines, etc.

The skull, consisting of twenty-two bones which form the head and face, contains the brain and organs of special sense—the eye, the ear, the nose and the tongue. The muscles of the face are small and numerous, with large and powerful muscles for mastication purposes.

The Spine or Vertebral Column is a flexible structure about two feet long, consisting of thirty-three vertebrae or separate segments of the backbone. These segments are named according to their position:

7 cervical vertebrae in the neck.

12 thoracic or dorsal vertebrae in the chest region.

5 lumbar vertebrae in the small of the back.

5 sacral vertebrae, fused together to form the sacrum, at the base of the spine.

4 coccygeal vertebrae forming the tail or coccyx.

These vertebrae move upon each other and are kept separate by means of thick pads of cartilage, called inter-vertebral discs, which give the whole backbone suppleness, deadening shocks and jars. Strong ligaments bind the vertebrae together.

The muscles of the back extend the length of the spinal column and on either side of it; their great size and strength are necessary for holding the body erect.

The Chest (Thorax) is a conical-shaped cavity made up of twelve vertebrae from which pass forward twelve ribs, curving around to the front of the body. These ribs enclose the chest and serve to protect the heart, lungs, liver, stomach, spleen, etc. The breast bone (sternum) is a flat bone lying at the front and middle of the chest.

The Upper Limb. The bones of the upper limb consist of:

The shoulder blade (scapula).
The collarbone (clavicle).
The bone of the upper arm (humerus).
The ulna $\Big\}$ bones of the forearm.
The radius
The 8 carpal bones $\Big\}$ bones of the wrist and hand.
The 5 metacarpal bones
The 14 phalanges

The upper end of the humerus forms a ball-and-socket joint with the shoulder blade, while its lower end forms the elbow joint with the upper ends of the radius and ulna; the former is on the thumb side of the arm and the latter on the inner or little finger side. Both bones reach from the elbow to the wrist, changing their relative positions with each turn of the hand.

The Hand is composed of the carpal bones, the metacarpal bones and the phalanges. The carpal bones are arranged in two rows of four and are the bones of the wrist; the metacarpal bones form the framework of the palm of the hand, and consist of five bones, each of which forms joints above with the carpal bones and below with the lower ends of the phalanges. The metacarpal bones form the knuckles, while the phalanges are the bones of the fingers and thumb, there being three phalanges in each finger and two in the thumb.

The Pelvis is a large basin-shaped mass of bone positioned between the lower end of the spine, which it supports, and the lower limbs on which it rests.

The Lower Limb. The bones of the lower limb are:

The thigh bone (femur).

The shin bone (tibia)
The splint bone (fibula) } bones of lower leg.

The kneecap (patella).

7 tarsal bones
5 metatarsal bones } bones of foot and ankle.
14 phalanges

The femur or thigh bone is the longest and strongest bone in the skeleton, as it has to take the weight of the whole body. It reaches from the hip joint to the knee joint, forming part of both joints. The kneecap or patella is a flat, almost triangular bone lying with its base uppermost, in front of the knee joint just below the surface of the skin. The shinbone or tibia is the strong bone extending from knee to ankle on the inside of the lower leg, while the fibula is the long, thin bone on the outside of the lower leg.

The Foot is composed of a group of seven irregular bones known as the tarsus, the metatarsus (five long bones in front of the tarsus, supporting the toes) and the phalanges or bones of the toes, of which there are two in the big toe and three in each of the outer toes.

### The Joints

A joint is formed at the junction where two or more bones meet, the surfaces of the bones which glide over each other to form the joints being covered by shining cartilage, which lessens friction. The majority of joints are freely movable, although those of the skull are immovable, while joints such as those between the vertebrae are slightly movable.

Movable joints are completely surrounded by strong fibrous tissue which forms an envelope, known as the capsule, containing the joint which is further strengthened by means of outside ligaments. The inside of a joint is lined with a delicate membrane, called the synovial membrane, which gives off a thick fluid known as synovial fluid. This acts as a lubricant allowing the cartilage-covered ends of bones to glide freely over each other.

There are four varieties of movable joints:

(a) Ball-and-Socket Joints consisting of a rounded head fitting into a hollow socket. Typical joints of this type are the hip joint and the shoulder joint. This type of joint allows movement in every direction.

(b) Hinge Joints. Movement is allowed only in one direction by this type of joint, that is hinge-like—forwards and backwards. The elbow and the joints between the metacarpal bones and the phalangeal bones of the hands are typical hinge joints. The knee joint is, of course, the principal hinge joint in the human body.

(c) Gliding Joints permit only very slight movement, one surface of the joint gliding over the other without any flexing or rotatory movement. The joints between the bones of the carpus of the hands and of the tarsus of the feet are examples.

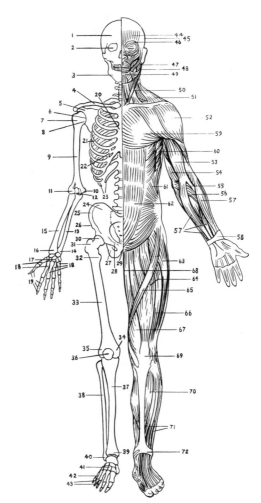

Fig. 21. Front View

## KEY TO DIAGRAM

### Representing The

### FRONT VIEW OF SKELETON AND MUSCLES

*Bones*

1. Cranium
2. Orbital fossa
3. Inferior maxilla
4. Clavicle
5. Coracoid Process of scapula
6. Head of humerus articulating with glenoid cavity of scapula
7. Greater tuberosity of humerus
8. Lesser tuberosity of humerus
9. Humerus
10. Internal condyle of humerus
11. External condyle of humerus
12. Coronoid process of ulna
13. Ulna
14. Styloid process of ulna
15. Radius
16. Styloid process of radius
17. Carpal bones
18. Metacarpal bones
19. Phalanges
20. Sternum
21. Ribs
22. Costal cartilages
23. Floating ribs
24. Ilium
25. Crest of ilium
26. Anterior superior spine of ilium
27. Ischium
28. Pubis
29. Symphysis pubis
30. Head of femur articulating with acetabulum
31. Greater trochanter of femur
32. Lesser trochanter of femur
33. Femur
34. Internal tuberosity of femur
35. External tuberosity of femur
36. Patella
37. Tibia
38. Fibula
39. Internal malleolus
40. External malleolus
41. Tarsal bones
42. Metatarsal bones.
43. Phalanges

*Muscles*

44. Occipitofrontalis, frontal part
45. Temporal
46. Orbicularis oculi
47. Zygomaticus
48. Masseter
49. Orbicularis oris
50. Sterno-mastoid
51. Trapezius
52. Deltoid
53. Biceps
54. Brachialis anticus
55. Tendon of biceps
56. Pronator radii teres
57. (Ulna side of forearm)—Flexors of wrist and digits (Radial side of forearm)—Brachioradialis
58. Annular ligament of wrist
59. Pectoralis major
60. Serratus magnus
61. Obliquus externus

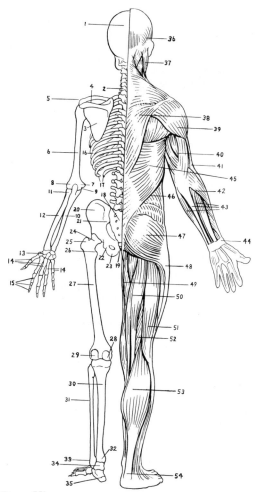

Fig. 22. Rear View

62. Sheath of rectus abdominis
63. Tensor fasciae latae
64. Rectus femoris
65. Sartorius
66. Vastus externus
67. Vastus internus
68. Adductors
69. Tendon of quadriceps extensor
70. Tibialis anticus
71. Extensors of toes
72. Annular ligament of ankle

## KEY TO DIAGRAM

### Representing The

### *REAR VIEW OF SKELETON AND MUSCLES*

#### *Bones*

1. Cranium
2. Vertebral column
3. Scapula
4. Spine of scapula
5. Acromion process of scapula
6. Humerus
7. Internal condyle of humerus
8. External condyle of humerus
9. Olecranon process of ulna
10. Ulna
11. Head of radius
12. Radius
13. Carpal bones
14. Metacarpal bones
15. Phalanges
16. Ribs
17. Floating ribs
18. Sacrum
19. Coccyx
20. Ilium
21. Posterior superior spine of ilium
22. Ischium
23. Tuberosity of ischium
24. Neck of femur
25. Greater trochanter of femur
26. Lesser trochanter of femur
27. Femur
28. Internal condyle of femur
29. External condyle of femur
30. Tibia
31. Fibula
32. Internal malleolus
33. External malleolus
34. Astragalus
35. Os Calcis

#### *Muscles*

36. Occipitofrontalis - occipital part
37. Sterno-mastoid
38. Trapezius
39. Deltoid
40. Triceps
41. Brachialis anticus
42. Brachio-radialis
43. Extensors of wrists and digits
44. Annular ligament of wrist
45. Latissimus dorsi
46. Obliquus externus
47. Gluteus maximus
48. Fascia lata
49. Gracilis
50. Semitendinosus
51. Biceps femoris
52. Semimembranosus
53. Gastrocnemius
54. Tendo-Achilles

(d) Pivot Joints. In this type of joint one bone forms a pivot around which the other bone rotates. The joints between the atlas and axis bones of the cervical part of the spine are examples; another example is the joint between the radius and the ulna bones.

There are certain technical terms used in dealing with the movements of joints, the use of which will give brevity and clarity to the description:

Flexion is the movement of bending a joint.

Extension is the movement of straightening a joint.

Abduction is the movement of drawing a limb away from the middle line of the body, as in lifting the arm away from the side of the body.

Adduction, the bringing of the limb towards the middle line of the body, as in returning the arm to the side following abduction.

Rotation, the turning of a joint on its own axis. This may be internal or external depending upon whether it is toward or away from the body.

Supination, the act of turning the palm of the hand away from the body by a movement of the radius bone over the ulna bone.

Pronation, the movement of turning the palm of the hand inward toward the body.

### The Muscular System

A muscle consists of a large number of fibers, covered and bound together by connective tissue, the whole being enclosed within a sheath. The sheath and the connective tissue inside the muscle are prolonged to form tendons of strong fibrous material at either end of the muscle. Each individual fiber is supplied with nerves and blood vessels, and has the power of contracting or relaxing under stimulation from the brain.

The body can move itself because of the motive power provided by its muscles. Energy is derived from the food that is eaten and stored in various parts of the body, to be released when required. This release takes the form of a highly complicated chemical combustion, resulting in contraction or relaxation of the muscle fibers, accompanied by the generation of heat. As the energy is used up by the muscles it is necessary for it to be replaced by a supply of oxygen and fuel conveyed by the blood. It is equally important that the waste products from chemical processes within the muscle are carried away by the blood.

The more "fixed" or stable part of the skeleton to which a muscle is attached is known as the Origin, and the more movable part is the Insertion; the origin is usually nearer the center of the body while the insertion is more distant. A shortening of the muscle in contraction will bring the origin and insertion closer together. Muscles which bend joints are called Flexors and those which straighten them are called Extensors— these are, of course, general terms.

When a man stands erect, his muscles are working to keep him upright or he would fall into a heap. Messages are passing constantly to the brain from the muscles that are stretched, from the skin of the soles of the feet and from those muscles which are tired. The brain works out all the messages and sends back impulses to keep other muscles at work. This process is unconscious, being automatic or reflex, because one is taught to stand up and walk from childhood. In order that the movements of the body will be well balanced, most of the muscle groups of the body are in pairs, the two having opposite actions. Thus it is possible to move a joint in both directions, very fine degrees of control being achieved by delicate adjustments of contraction and relaxation in the respective groups.

It is not necessary for the teacher, or indeed the dancer herself, to be conversant with all the two hundred or so muscles of the human body, nor for her to learn all the refinements of their actions and structure. If some degree of basic familiarity is obtained with the main muscles responsible for the fundamental movements of the body, particularly those used in each particular activity, it will be adequate for their purposes.

The Principal Muscles of the Body

(1) *Acting on the Head and Neck*
  (a) *Muscles of mastication*
      Temporal
      Masseter
  (b) *Bending forward of head (Flexion)*
      Rectus capitis anticus
      Longus colli
  (c) *Bending backwards of head (Extension)*
      Upper part of erector spinae
  (d) *Side flexion of head*
      Sternomastoid
      Scaleni

(2) *Muscles of the Trunk*
  (a) *Bending backwards of the spine (Extension)*
      Erector spinae
  (b) *Bending forwards of the spine (Flexion)*
      ABDOMINAL MUSCLES:
      Rectus abdominis

External abdominal oblique
Internal abdominal oblique
Transversalis
(c) *Side flexion of the spine*
Quadratus lumborum
(3) *Muscles of the Upper Extremity.*
    (a) *Raising of shoulder girdle*
    Trapezius
    Levator anguli scapulae
    (b) *Lowering or depression of shoulder girdle.*
    Serratus magnus
    (c) *Pulling shoulders forward (Abduction)*
    Serratus magnus
    (d) *Bracing shoulders back (Adduction)*
    Trapezius (middle fibers)
    Rhomboids (major & minor)
    (e) *Flexion of the shoulder joint*
    Pectoralis major
    Deltoid
    Biceps
    Coracobrachialis
    (f) *Extension of shoulder joint (drawing arm back)*
    Deltoid (middle and rear fibers)
    Pectoralis major
    Latissimus dorsi
    Teres major
    (g) *Lifting arm away from side of body (Abduction)*
    Deltoid
    Supraspinatus
    (h) *Lowering arm to side of body (Adduction)*
    Pectoralis major

Latissimus dorsi
Teres major

(i) *Inwardly rotating the arm*
Pectoralis major
Deltoid (front fibers)
Latissimus dorsi
Teres major
Subscapularis

(j) *Outwardly rotating the arm*
Deltoid (rear fibers)
Teres minor
Infraspinatus

(4) *Muscles Acting on the Elbow Joint*

(a) *Bending the elbow (Flexion)*
Brachialis anticus
Biceps

(b) *Straightening the elbow (Extension)*
Triceps

(c) *Turning palm of hand downwards (Pronation)*
Pronator radii teres
Pronator quadratus

(d) *Turning palm of hand upwards (Supination)*
Biceps
Supinator brevis

(5) *Muscles Acting on the Wrist, Fingers and Thumb*

(a) *Bending the wrist (Flexion)*
Flexors of the wrist

This comprises a group of muscles attached to a common point on the inside of the elbow joint, and passing downwards on the front of the forearm.

(b) *Straightening the wrist (Extension)*

Extensors of the wrist

This comprises a group of muscles working from a common point on the outside of the elbow joint, and passing downwards on the back of the forearm.

      (c) *Bending the fingers (Flexion)*
          As in (a) above
      (d) *Straightening the fingers (Extension)*
          As in (b) above

(6) *Muscles of the Lower Extremity.*

      (a) *Bending the hip joint (Flexion)*
          Ilio-psoas
          Rectus femoris
      (b) *Straightening the hip joint (Extension)*
          Gluteus maximus
          Hamstrings
      (c) *Lifting the leg sideways (Abduction)*
          Gluteus medius
          Gluteus minimus
      (d) *Returning the leg to the midline (Adduction)*
          Adductor magnus
          Adductor longus
          Adductor brevis
      (e) *Outward rotation of the leg*
          Adductor muscles
          Obturators
      (f) *Inward rotation of the leg*
          Gluteus medius

(7) *Muscles Acting on the Knee Joint*

      (a) *Bending the knee (Flexion)*
          Hamstrings
          Gastrocnemius
          Soleus

(b) *Straightening the knee (Extension)*
Quadriceps Group—composed of
Rectus femoris
Vastus externus
Vastus internus
Vastus intermedius
(8) *Muscles Acting on the Foot and Ankle.*
(a) *Pulling the foot and toes upwards
(Dorsi-flexion)*
Tibialis anticus
Extensor muscles
(b) *Pointing the foot and toes downwards
(Plantar-flexion)*
Gastrocnemius
Soleus
Tibialis posticus
Peroneus longus
Flexor muscles

## *PHYSIOLOGY*

### *How the Human Body Works*

One of the aims of physical education, sport and rec-
reation is to assist in the normal growth and development of the human body, and the maintenance of a certain
degree of physical fitness. For this, a knowledge of physiology is essential. Every dancer will have noticed the
powerful effect of muscular activity on the processes of
her body. The breathing speeds up and becomes deeper,
the heart beats faster, she feels warmer, and perspiration becomes noticeable. These changes indicate that
certain adjustments have been made in order to mobilize

the human organism for a greater output of energy. It is important that those in charge of dancers, just as much as athletes, have a basic knowledge of these changes, that they are aware that nerves must stimulate muscles to contract, that fuel must be made available for the muscles and other organs, that oxygen has to be provided and waste products eliminated.

### The Cardiovascular System

The cardiovascular system consists of the blood and the organs of circulation, which are as follows:

The Heart which pumps the blood around the body.

The Arteries through which runs the blood from the heart.

The Veins through which runs the blood returning to the heart.

The Capillaries form a network of hairlike vessels throughout the body which communicate with the arteries and veins to permit the exchange of gases, food and waste products with the tissues.

The Lymphatics are minute vessels of a nature similar to the capillaries and run throughout the same parts of the body. They have valves which permit the one-way passage back to the blood stream of the plasma-part of the blood, which has passed out through the walls of the capillaries and flooded the tissues of the body.

The arteries divide into branches, which become gradually smaller by repeated subdivision, until they finally end as capillaries. The blood in the arteries is under the high pressure given to it by the force of the heart beat; for this reason when an artery is cut, blood spurts out of it. The veins are the vessels along which blood is carried back to the heart; if they are cut, blood only wells out of them in a steady stream, and is dark in color. The tissues of the body are nourished by the circulating blood, and by means of this blood waste materials are also carried from the tissues to the excretory organs of the body so that they may be eliminated from the system. It is essential to life that blood should remain fluid within the vessels, yet become clotted when shed and in contact with the air. The maintenance of this fluidity is essential for the circulation of the blood, while clotting provides an important defense against excessive bleeding from wounds.

The total quantity of blood contained in the body varies at different times, but it may be estimated on the average at not less than one-twentieth or about 5 percent of the weight of the body. Its distribution may be stated in round numbers as follows:

One-quarter in the heart, lungs and large blood vessels.
One-quarter in the liver.
One-quarter in the muscles of the body.
One-quarter in the other organs of the body.

As a general summary of the circulation, the blood leaves the heart via the aorta (a large blood vessel) and is pumped all over the body; that which goes to the spleen, stomach and the intestines is taken to the liver and then back to the inferior vena cava (this is known as the portal circulation). The remainder returns to the right auricle (chamber) of the heart, via the systemic veins, ending in the venae cavae (the systemic circulation). Except for the pulmonary arteries and veins, the arteries carry pure, oxygenated bright red blood, and the veins carry impure, dark blood.

## The Respiratory System

The respiratory system is formed by the respiratory passages—the nose, mouth, throat (pharynx), voice box (larynx), windpipe (trachea) and the lungs. The pharynx (throat) is the cavity at the back of the nose and mouth, and is the channel through which food and air pass downwards, the air passing via the larynx. The windpipe (trachea) is a short, wide tube which is held open by rings of cartilage, eventually dividing into two major branches which pass to each of the two lungs. After entering the lungs they divide and subdivide to form minute tubes throughout the lungs. The lungs are greyish, spongy organs, conical in shape, lying on each side of the heart and above the diaphragm in the two sides of the chest cavity. The right lung is divided into three lobes, the left into two lobes.

Respiration or breathing is the process of drawing air into the lungs (inspiration) and expelling it (expiration) so that an interchange of gases between the air and the blood may take place. Inspiration is a muscular effort, while expiration requires no effort as the muscles relax, the size of the chest cavity is reduced and the lungs recoil to their smallest size.

During its passage around the body, the blood gives up to the tissues the oxygen it contained on leaving the heart, and at the same time it absorbs moisture and carbon dioxide, which gives the dark blue colour. The blood then returns to the heart, passing through it to the lungs. In the small capillary vessels of the lungs it gives up the moisture and carbon dioxide and absorbs oxygen from the tissues of the lungs, thus gaining a bright red color.

It is now ready to recirculate around the body, taking nourishment to all parts.

It is possible to measure the ventilation power of the lungs; the sum of the various air stocks in the lungs being known as vital capacity. Vital capacity varies in different individuals and can be greatly improved by suitable exercises and sports, the greater the vital capacity in proportion to height, weight, etc., the better the performance of the dancer.

## The Nervous System

Nervous tissue consists of nerve cells and nerve fibers; the cells generate and receive impulses, the fibers only transmit the impulses. It is through nervous tissue that the different parts of the body communicate, and it is the means by which the body keeps in touch with the outside world. The cells are highly specialized, but pay for this specialization by lacking the ability to reproduce themselves. Once destroyed they cannot be regenerated. The nervous system is divided into three parts:

The central nervous system.

The nerves themselves.

The autonomic nervous system.

The central nervous system consists of the brain and the spinal cord. The former acts as the counterpart of a telephone exchange in that it receives information via the incoming nerves, acts on this knowledge when necessary through the outgoing nerves and may finally store up useful facts in the memory.

The nerves can be classified as cranial or spinal according to their positions. The cranial nerves are given off from the brain in pairs, twelve in number. They supply the organs of special sense, the skin and the muscles of the face, the heart, lungs, and the stomach. The spinal nerves are thirty-one pairs in number and are given off in pairs from descending levels of the spine. All the power of causing muscular contraction which a spinal nerve possesses is lodged in the fibers which compose the front (or anterior) nerve roots, and all the power of giving rise to sensation, in those of the rear (or posterior) nerve roots. Hence the anterior nerve roots are commonly called "motor" and the posterior nerve roots "sensory." Motor nerves control the action of voluntary muscles, the will to make the movement originating in the brain. Sensory nerves enter the spinal cord by the posterior nerve roots and convey to the brain the sensation of touch, heat, cold, pain and pressure. The nerves of sight, smell, taste and hearing are also sensory nerves, entering the brain directly.

The spinal cord possesses a peculiar power of receiving a stimulation or impulse from an outside source and, without transmitting that message to the brain, of causing a muscular movement in response to that impulse. This is known as a reflex action.

The autonomic nervous system is used to regulate the involuntary movements and functions of the body, such as the circulation and breathing. It works quite independently of the brain, continuing during sleep and unconsciousness.

### The Digestive System

Digestion is the process of breaking down food into substances which may be absorbed into the body. The system by which this takes place is known as the digestive system and is composed of the alimentary canal and the accessory organs.

The alimentary canal is a long tube beginning at the mouth and ending at the anus, the composite parts consisting of the mouth, throat, gullet, stomach, small and large intestines. The accessory organs are the teeth, tongue, salivary glands, gastric and intestinal glands, liver and pancreas.

It is not within the scope of this volume to discuss food and diet, save to say that food is necessary for growth, to replace wear and tear, and to supply warmth and energy. It consists of protein, carbohydrates and fats, mineral salts, vitamins and water. The chemical processes of the body during life are known as metabolism.

# *PART II*
# THE PREVENTION OF INJURY

# 2

# Factors in the Prevention of Injuries

Anyone who takes part in strenuous physical activities runs the risk of sustaining an injury at one time or another, and this applies equally to ballet dancing as to tennis, athletics or, perhaps with greater risks, the body-contact sports such as football, rugger, etc. Some of these injuries begin long before the dancer finds it impossible to take another step without pain or to jump with her normal ease and grace. These injuries are initiated with an apparently insignificant occurrence, momentarily painful, which subsides and leaves few noticeable reactions. Later, through neglect or incorrect treatment, the condition becomes a relatively serious injury. On the other hand, the injury may violently arrive by the sudden accidental collision of bodies, or through a slip of the foot that brings a dancer crashing to the floor. On these occasions, one usefully remembers that there is nothing more irretrievable than an accident!

No factor is more important in the prevention of injury than physical fitness and physical training.

Mankind has necessarily been interested in physical fitness since the days of the cave man, as a means of actual survival because only the fittest men could live under the primitive conditions prevailing, and only the fittest men could hunt to provide the food essential for life.

Only during the last fifty years has there been any real understanding of the actual physiological factors involved in the question of physical fitness, but much has been done during this period.

An accurate definition of physical fitness is the development of the body to a state so that a given amount of physical work can be produced, when required, with a minimum of physical effort. This obviously requires the greatest physical efficiency, and is dependent upon the mutual development of the various bodily systems, such as the muscular, respiratory, circulatory, coordinated by the central nervous system. There are three processes involved:

(a) The muscular changes necessary for energy production.

(b) Adjustments in the circulatory and respiratory systems to remove waste products and provide the muscles with oxygen and foodstuffs.

(c) The means of coordination.

We all know of those "born" athletes who spring from triumph to triumph with few apparent physical attributes rendering them different from their fellow men. The reason for their successes is in their coordinating mechanism, making the various bodily systems "click" in such a fashion as to render them superior to their opponents. Only a very small proportion of mankind possess this great gift, but it is possible for the average athlete to compensate for that lack by means of planned physical training.

The great importance of physical exercise lies in the fact that by carefully graduated training, it is possible to develop the muscles to a stage of actual energy production more than three times the normal rate. At the same time there will be a 400 percent increase in the number of capillaries and 100 percent increase in their size. Bodily fitness is attained by training, the aims of which are to be light, agile, perform movements easily with economy of effort and to have complete control over the entire body. Training develops strength, speed, agility, skill, endurance, flexibility, balance, reaction time and it also controls the body weight.

The part played by fitness in the prevention of injury causes the muscles to possess tone and strength, sufficient to support the joints on which they work, and to protect them from stress and strain. The improvement in "reaction time" brought on by training is also important in that it improves the dancer's sense of rhythm and timing. In this way the dancer can automatically "come in" or commence a movement at precisely the right moment so that she entails a minimum of risk. Reaction time can be explained by a recent experiment in America. The players of a leading baseball club sat in front of complicated timing apparatus, controlled by a pressbutton, which had to be operated each time a red-light signal was flashed high on the wall. In every case the apparatus timed the players with the quickest reactions as being first team men, and presumably fitter and more skilled athletes. The acquisition of speed in the footballer, for example, is emphasized by the fact that wingers, who are probably the speediest men in a team, are also the least often injured.

Once a general fitness foundation has been built up by a planned and graduated program of physical exercise, it is then possible to teach skills and techniques, the acquisition of which obviously renders an artiste better fitted to fight off injury. The training involved in this building of a fitness foundation will also give strength and tone to the vital muscle groups, enabling the excessive strain of activity to be borne by the muscle and not by the ligaments, which are inelastic structures not constructed for such work.

A dancing class possesses one unique injury-prevention factor—almost a "built-in" asset, in fact! Athletes are advised, often fruitlessly, to include in their training schedule routines of exercises designed to strengthen the more frequently injured muscle groups. But a dancer appears to have a most adequate routine of this nature embodied in her normal warming-up and limbering exercises. These exercises will also strengthen the ligaments supporting the joints upon which the muscles work. All muscles of the legs, for example, should be strengthened, and should also be put through a daily routine which ensures that they are all stretched to their limit. Muscles which are accustomed to being stretched will not so readily tear when exposed to sudden stress through a violent stretching. These preventative-type exercises will, of course, also fulfill the physiological requirements of any normal exercise routine.

Recurrent injuries are the bane of the dancer's life just as they are to the athlete. They arise from an initial injury which has been neglected or incorrectly treated, thus creating a weak link in the physical chain.

These old chronic painful conditions occur frequently in the ankles, groins and knees and are extremely difficult to treat. In spite of the most conscientious treatment it will often be necessary to have the dancer manipulated by a surgeon, under anaesthetic, to break down the limiting and painful adhesions. No dancer with a history of a weakened joint should be permitted to take part in prolonged and strenuous practices without adequate strapping, which will protect and support the joint, thus preventing aggravation of the injury. But to rely solely on this strapping is the height of folly and more than optimistic; the muscle tone and strength must be restored to the muscle groups around the joint so that they take their proper part in supporting the joint. It is essential never to relax completely when performing because heavy thrusts and strains striking a relaxed person will injure an old sprained joint, even with strapping in place.

An athlete, and similarly a dancer, might well be more likely to sustain injury during the later stages of a game (or a performance) because he (or she) is less on their subconscious guard against shock owing to fatigue. On the other hand, by this stage the body will be so warmed up as to be in the best physical condition to withstand an injury. It is interesting to note that the author's observations indicate that injuries generally occur in students carrying out major work. Through overenthusiasm; "pushing" for examinations or with professional ambitions, these students "overextend."

On the more material side of injury prevention—and more responsive to human agencies—is the room or studio in which classes are held. Here, in this large room, lie many hazards for the unwary dancer; luckily a little care and foresight can eliminate most of them.

*The Floor:* Ideally the floor should be wooden and smooth without being slippery. Of course, there must be no splinters.

*The Bar:* Must not be *too* firm otherwise pupils begin to rely too much upon it. Some bars lift out when they are pulled up; this has certain disadvantages. Russian studios often have bars that are heavily weighted or firmly set into the wall. This enables the dancers to obtain maximum support.

*Lighting:* Must be good and adequate for the size of the room. The recommendations of experts on lighting can be obtained without too much difficulty.

*Space:* Ideally, the room should be square and sufficiently large to avoid crowding and subsequent body contact. Conversely, the numbers of pupils in a class should be governed by the size of the studio.

*Heating:* The studio must be reasonably warm without being stuffy. If it is cold, it takes too long to warm up or else the warm-up period is insufficient to prevent injury. All forms of heating appliances should be adequately protected so as to avoid burns through contact; they should also be regularly inspected and serviced.

*Ventilation:* Must be adequate and free from drafts.

*Equipment:* Should be regularly checked and serviced to ensure firm fixing and be free from faults.

# 3

# The Teacher's Role in Injury Prevention

The principal role of the teacher of dancing is to draw from each individual pupil the best possible results— working within their specific capabilities and in SAFETY. She must "feel movement" and impart that knowledge to her pupils. Dancers are athletes—and all athletes are injury-prone. It is the duty of every teacher to ensure that her charges possess a reasonable standard of physical fitness, sufficient to fight off the more common injuries. She must take all possible steps to prevent injuries both in practice and in actual performance. But, even in the best ordered circles, accidents can happen, and it is essential for the teacher to have sufficient basic knowledge to treat an injury correctly, safely and as quickly as possible.

Experience has shown that in the world of sport a large proportion of injuries can be prevented or minimized with adequate supervision and foresight. It is reasonable to claim that the same situation applies to the world of dancing. Injury is the occupational hazard of most forms of physical activity; physical fitness and training are its direct opponents.

A good teacher working in a barn could train pupils

to higher standards than a bad teacher working in the most sumptuous modern studio. Primarily, this is because a good teacher has, above everything else, the right sort of personality and temperament. She realizes, perhaps innately, that firm leadership and supervision is essential; that injury-producing situations are prevented by personality, example and the sensible use of authority. She knows when to be stern and severe, yet she is always just and fair; she has no favorites and, because she knows her job from A to Z, her pupils respect her.

As far as injury prevention is concerned, there are certain precepts which every teacher must observe:

(1) A teacher must drill all pupils to report injuries to her. The minor, unattended injury of today is the disabling major injury of tomorrow.

(2) A teacher must possess a trained sense of judgement as to the gravity of an injury so that she knows when it is safe to allow a pupil to dance or when to order a halt.

(3) It is debatable whether the dedicated dancer finds ANY part of her training to be boring or monotonous, but all pupils are not fired with the same enthusiasm! Therefore, the teacher must insist that those less-interesting parts of training are carried out as conscientiously as are the more interesting features. This particularly applies to the open "warming-up" session.

(4) Where injury prevention is concerned, it is an advantage for the teacher to be able to assess the personality and character of the dancer in addition to being familiar with the demands made upon her. Such knowledge is also useful in evaluating the severity of an injury; so variable is human nature that an injury can be to one dancer a major disaster while another

dancer of different temperament will view it only as a minor irritation!

The dancer herself has a vital part to play; along with her teacher she must remember that all dancing movements are not a matter for muscles alone but must be based on the deep bony structure of the human body. This has been excellently postulated by Celia Sparger, a Member of the Chartered Society of Physiotherapy and a ballet lover who is also highly experienced in the prevention and treatment of dancing injuries. In her book "Anatomy and Ballet" (A. and C. Black, London, 1949) Miss Sparger writes:

"If the movements are performed correctly the correct muscles will work."

Therefore, she advocates that one must see the moving body as a moving skeleton so that the natural relationship of the bones and the limitations of their movements can be fully appreciated. If both pupil and teacher follow this reasoning it should go a long way toward preventing injury to the delicate apparatus by which the art of dance is created. The dancer should possess (her teacher should ensure that she has, and encourage it) an intelligent knowledge of what she is physically doing in each exercise. The pupil should not work mechanically; ideally, she should have a basic knowledge of the muscles, joints and bones concerned.

There is a need for painstaking planning so that teaching, particularly that of an elementary routine, is slow and gradual; that it is graded and adapted to cope with the inevitable differences in physical size and capabilities. To a certain extent, the laid-down syllabus of the various examining bodies cater to this. It is in the early stages that initial mistakes have to be eliminated so that they do not become ingrained and difficult to eradicate later. More than that, it is essential that no pupil should ever get hurt attempting to carry out a movement or exercise beyond her physical capabilities. Grace, vitality and vigor can, at times, dangerously disguise faults but an imperfect dancer can be injured in trying to extend her scope. Only a step-by-step technique can give a safe mastery of the art.

To point out a dangerous mistake is not enough; the pupil may be too young to understand; only the teacher can spot the cause of the mistake and find the remedy. To merely order a revised repetition of the step or movement is inadequate; the offending movement should be analytically dissected and a specific exercise given to that particular set of muscles or the joint that is not working correctly. Such methods of training must be sustained efforts but not forced ones. A pupil must NEVER be permitted to become dangerously fatigued attempting to carry out an exercise beyond her physical ability.

A dangerous, injury-producing fault can be due either to lack of attention, to lack of strength or to a physical shortcoming. Each of these cases requires a different method of correction. Backwardness and lack of attention have their own "built-in" injury-producing qualities; a psychological approach is required on the part of the teacher. In fact, an insight into pupils' psychology is essential to a teacher. Lack of physical strength can be remedied by devising appropriate exercises to give extra work to the weaker muscles.

A teacher must possess the faculty to determine the cause of an obstinate fault or a fault that can produce an injury. If it is due to a physical shortcoming, the pupil will only become exasperated by repeated chiding and will not improve. A child with a disability or a lack of ideal features must never be permitted to enthusiastically overwork to overcome these handicaps. This must not be confused with one of the many physical defects due more to stiffness of muscle rather than to any physical malformation; these cases will respond to planned limbering exercises. A specific case is that of insufficient stretching power of the "hamstring" muscles behind the knee. It is probably beyond the pupil's power to stretch the knees unless she is helped to get rid of the defect which is preventing her from stretching them.

The majority of injuries occur for trivial and easily explained reasons, particularly those which take place during practice or teaching. Such examples spring to mind of the tiring pupil who is given a new round of strenuous movements toward the end of a practice session, perhaps by a new and fresh teacher. Obviously, a class will progressively tire as the work proceeds; if more than one teacher is taking them then the injury-prone situation occurs where the rapidly tiring pupils are assailed by the fresh teacher.

Warming up is so vital as to merit a section of its own; one facet however can be considered at this stage. A class will chill while watching the demonstration of some more complicated movements so that when their turn to perform eventually comes they are in a dangerously cold condition. When demonstrations are being given, a class should warm up again before being called upon for physical stress. Admittedly, this rarely occurs, pauses are usually only long enough for the breath to be regained.

The teacher must ensure that no dancer performs any straining or strenuous movements until she is 100 percent fit after an injury—better to have a fit under-study than an unfit star who will break down in the middle of a performance!

With adequate training and supervision by their teachers, dancers can focus their full attention on technical ability and on the physical, mental and financial benefits that dancing can bring to them, rather than on the bogey of possible crippling injuries. By conforming to these ideals, years can be added to the performing, and natural lives of the dancers concerned.

# 4

# Appearance and its Effect on Injury Prevention

Both on the sports field and on the stage, the performer who "looks" good is usually the one who is doing the job properly. She is using the skill and technique derived from training, coupled with natural ability, to produce a performance that pleases. It follows that if an artiste looks good (if it is accepted that looking good means to be performing in accordance with high standards) then it is reasonable to assume that she is performing safely, in a manner unlikely to cause injury. In this way, the aesthetic and the practical aspects of physical activity are coupled together. Bearing in mind this relationship of appearance plus efficiency leads to safety in dancing, let us work on an anatomical survey that will throw the relevant factors into correct perspective.

The whole is more than the sum of its parts: by physically improving the separate sections of the body a perfect whole can be built. A dancer is produced for what she looks like from the front; the aim is an audience-pleasing view. Obviously, this means that the silhouette as a whole is the first thing that catches the eye when a dancer makes her entrance. This silhouette should be compact and neat—a small head carried well; slim neck; a back that is straight but not too tense or rigid; shoulders pressed down and not too square, for this gives a masculine appearance; small bust; arms well-balanced and relaxed sufficiently to give an attractive line; small waist; long slim legs moving easily from the hips. ADAGE movements are generally performed better by a long-legged dancer, possibly because of control over length of leg; a short-legged dancer is better at BATTERIE. The hips must also be slim, for they lengthen the line of the legs; an effect of length is essential to the silhouette. The feet must move smoothly and easily. Height —not too tall—five feet four inches is ideal; a tall girl will find it difficult to obtain partners and, on stage, one tends to look bigger than in life.

The well-balanced whole affects not only the appearance and performance, but also the "injury proneness" of the dancer. Therefore work and exercises giving and encouraging this coordinated balance must be constantly practiced; it is achieved in the practice of the ADAGE and the ENCHAINEMENTS of ALLEGRO. The more balanced and compact the dancer is in herself, the easier is her body to guide and control through these practices. At all times, it must be remembered that it is the correlation of the extremities that take precedence over the trunk.

To obtain the necessary balance and coordination, limbering exercises are required in addition to the usual technical practices. All beauty of line and form depends upon suppleness, as a tense and rigid body will never have balance or carriage. It is necessary for a dancer to be supple before any great corrective or technical effort can be made; in addition, suppleness greatly aids in preventing injury. In this connection, it is interesting to note that boys generally lack suppleness because the male skeleton is not naturally pliable enough. If, in the formative period, boys lose suppleness altogether, then their ARABESQUES lack beauty of line, the back has no curve and jumps are ugly. Boys should be encouraged to do limbering and stretching exercises; carefully and only when adequately warmed up.

All movements and exercises of relaxation using the whole body are good. For example;

(1) Rolling from side to side on the floor; an exercise that is very effective in slimming the hips.

(2) Big body swings taken in a standing posture.

Good carriage is aided by exercises which contract both the abdominal and lumbar muscles. The waist is the pivot of the body and the center of balance; keep it slim and supple by practicing movements that turn the body above the pelvis. Stretch up, with arms above the head as though trying to pick an almost-out-of-reach apple from a tree, using first one hand then the other, rising onto the toes. The same type of exercise taken with a side stretch can be done with a partner. Standing about six inches out of each other's reach, sustain the side-bend with arms stretched parallel above the head until each partner can grasp the other's fingers.

"Forced limbering" must never be done. This includes pupils limbering each other by grasping legs and forcing their normal limit, in second position or in Arabesque. Pupils should only limber as far as they are physically able without outside help.

Posture and carriage are inextricably bound together. Bad posture acquired during rudimentary training has ruined the chances of entry into the Royal Ballet School of many young dancers. Dame Ninette de Valois, in this connection, has written:

"Incorrect posture, irrespective of technical standard, might become the main reason for a child failing to obtain any examination "pass." Good teachers are not always able to remedy this defect in later years, and it is necessary that we rid ourselves of this increasing menace."

The legs are the key that opens the door to a dancer's career; they are the first thing which a manager looks at during an audition. Their care and conditioning, together with their preservation, should be one of the chief concerns of the student. Beauty of line and form must disguise the strength that is possessed by strong and shapely legs. Unless the legs are well-porportioned, straight and well-shaped it is useless for their owner to hope for a dancer's career. Many would-be dancers' souls languish in a body supported by legs that are bandy, knock-kneed or which bulge in front! Well-proportioned legs should not be too long in the thigh, or too short from knee to ankle—similarly the body must not be too long and carried on legs that are too short.

The legs need continual exercise because they are the most heavily muscled parts of the body; exercise practiced with discrimination will ensure that they do not become overdeveloped. If practiced too much, GRANDS BATTEMENTS, for example, tend to overdevelop the thighs in children and young students. Do not overdo the leg work; get the body weight off the legs by practicing leg work lying on the floor. Use the breathing to lighten the poise of the body—it should not sag into the hips so that it is a dead weight on the legs. Lift up from the pelvis without raising the shoulders. It is from the lower abdominal muscles that most of the strength in leg work comes; many dancers try to take all their strength from the legs, both in BATTEMENTS and elevation; the lower abdominal and back muscles should also play their part. The trunk is vitally instrumental in perfecting leg work; limbering exercises which tone up and loosen the whole body can also lengthen the legs.

This chapter is basically aimed at the young dancer; however it is not inapplicable to conclude with a word of advice to teachers on the subject of legs. Teachers and choreographers have to demonstrate the work they require; legs that did hard work in student days become neglected when the practical work lessens. They are apt to become thick and heavy, liable to cramp and other troublesome conditions arising from muscular devitalization. If the legs begin to get out of hand in this way rest them as much as possible with the feet up, getting the weight off them. Give them gentle and regular exercise with perhaps a little massage.

# 5

# Posture and Injury Prevention

Posture and dance training are inextricably interwoven; the latter brings immeasurable benefits to the former but, in its turn, is to a certain extent dependent upon it. A trained dancer stands out in a crowd; her movements and positions are graceful and poised albeit slightly tinged with the theater! Dancing encourages muscular extension, a characteristic of human adult posture; it is interesting to reflect that the emotions of joy, pride and happiness all express themselves in postures of bodily extension and not in cramped flexion.

There are innumerable concepts of human posture with many interpretations of its significance, it is "all things to all men"—it may be a racial characteristic, an indication of the soundness of one's skeletal framework and muscular system, an expression of personality and emotions, an expression of mood or character. The surgeon, the physical educationalist, the artist, the physician, the biologist, the model, the employer, the sculptor, the dancer—all see posture within the framework of their own profession and interest.

Poor posture prevents the body from functioning properly because a part or parts are out of alignment, this causes mechanical readjustment resulting in muscular effort and in strain. Many authorities such as Schneider and Karpovich, Laplace and Nicholson among others, have stated that improvements in posture have given no scientific proof of definite improvements in the physiological functions of the body. Tests on twenty-three subjects, after having their posture corrected, showed very little improvement in circulatory efficiency and, after a year, only eight had maintained their postural correction. The passing of time had not apparently made them any more efficient physiologically. Poor posture is said to contribute to decreased lung capacity, poor circulation, irregular elimination and general lowering of health standards, but there is no scientific proof of these statements. Therefore, if one is to accept that postural standards should be improved, such improvement can only be carried out on the grounds of preventing physical strain and its effects.

It is, perhaps, the teachers of dancing who form the staunchest defenders against those "Posture Enthusiasts" who wish to flatten the low-back curve on aesthetic grounds. Such people are sadly affecting the mobility of the spine which, with the exception of rotation, is greatest in the lumbar or low-back region where the curve is normally concave. When this curve is structurally increased or decreased the movements of the spine in this area are affected. The reasons for mobility being affected lie in the fact that it is controlled by the thickness of the intervertebral disc, by the plane of the articular surfaces of the vertebral joints, by the tightness or laxness of spinal ligaments and by muscular tension.

People with perfectly straight spinal columns are often seen; they do not necessarily suffer any disability and are generally considered to carry themselves well. It cannot be denied, as already quoted, that a straight back gives an agreeable posture from an aesthetic point of view, whereas an exaggerated low-back curve leads to prominence of the belly and buttocks. This leads to the apparently logical opinion that the low-back curve should be as slight in degree as possible. But the inward curves in the low-back area and in the neck have been developed in order to protect the intervertebral discs in those areas from excessive strain! The vertebrae most likely to suffer disc displacement are the fourth, sixth and seventh cervical (in the neck) and the fourth and fifth lumbar (in the lower back) and they are the very areas of the spine where the curve is most marked. Interestingly, these curves are absent at birth and during the first year of extra-uterine life, so their development must be recent and connected with man's adoption of the erect posture.

The existence of these curves means that the space between the vertebrae named above is wider in front than at the back, thus a slight pressure is maintained on the disc in that space, in a forward direction, during weight-bearing. People with flat backs have not such protection for their discs and it is noticeable that such people are more likely to suffer from backache, because their joint surfaces lie parallel when they stand upright so that even the slightest forward flexion of the spine at once begins to squeeze their discs backwards. People with a normal or exaggerated low-back curve have to bend well forward before the back of the joint between the vertebrae is wider than the front. On such simple facts, is borne the whole case for sensible posture. If a person with a flat lower back has a tendency toward backache the mechanics of the movement within the vertebral joint means that even the smallest degree of stooping will cause pain through movement of the disc, but the person with backache who possesses normal low-back curves will be able to bend quite happily providing he doesn't go forward further than the mid-position.

If these facts are accepted then it is evident that much harm can come from the misdirected exercises normally given in posture training. Such exercises should never include trunk-flexion and no effort should be made to flatten the lower back. In other words, postural exercises must be guided by the prevention of future backache and not aesthetic principles. *

A posture is any momentarily stationary attitude the body assumes. Every activity is really a series of attitudes which differ in sport, work and everyday life and which may be mechanically efficient or they may subject the body to strain. Many of the postures of our daily occupations and recreations could well be analyzed in the interests of improved output with less effort and less static injury. Part of the difficulty in laying down postural principles is due to the fact that no individual's posture can be adequately described. Posture means position but must not imply merely standing or sitting erect because a multi-segmented organism such as the human body cannot be said to have a single position. Good posture in a human being is dynamic, not static, and means that the body assumes many postures and rarely holds any of them for an appreciable time. All postures need balanced action of muscles to maintain them in positions which do not involve undue strain and from which immediate coordinated action of any part of the body is

* It must be recorded that Rona Allen, F. I. S. T. D. (N. D. B. Comm), L. I. S. T. D. (I. S. B.) technical advisor to the author, profoundly disagrees with these views! She states: "These conclusions are contrary to everything I teach and believe to be right."

possible. It is difficult, if not impossible, to measure or even record characteristic postural patterns although the occupational characteristics of many people are distinctly revealed in their normal walking, sitting and resting positions because the relative development of muscles is determined by day-to-day usage.

It takes practice and observation to adequately evaluate posture; there are no foolproof rule-of-thumb measurements which will give an adequate analysis of posture. A patient's age, sex, physical attributes and occupation must be considered. Generally speaking, it is necessary to observe bodily balance or alignment, position of the head, depth of spinal curves and level of the shoulders. The observer is aided by man's unique capacity for accuracy of movement, due to his upright position, the adaption of some of his muscles for stabilizing postural work and others for quick, accurate active work, and the higher development of controlling nerve centers. Many lower animals such as the dog, the ape or the cat, are more supple than the average human being but lack his capacity for accurate movement.

The human skeleton is wonderfully adapted for the many active functions that it has to fulfill, but it can only be maintained in the erect position by vigilant action of the muscles controlling it, and good posture takes less muscular effort to maintain than poor posture. The main contributing factor in chronic strain of the lower back is poor muscular control or poor body mechanics. For example, when the normal low-back curve is eliminated the body's center of gravity is forward of its normal plane and the spinal muscles are subject to greater strain which, if long continued, will result in back pain. There are certain principles related to the mechanism for maintaining and adjusting erect posture. Stimuli arising from vision, from the balancing mechanisms of the ears, from muscular stretching and pressure on the soles of the feet, provide the body with a means of remaining upright without the necessity of conscious control. By the same means, temporary postural adjustments can be made. The cost in energy of standing posture seems to be smallest in a posture where the knees are braced back to their maximum, the hips are pushed forward to the limit, the curve of the upper back is increased to the maximum, the head is projected forward and the upper trunk is inclined slightly backward. This, of course, represents a typical picture of fatigue posture and a common variation of it is a shift of the weight to one foot with accompanying asymmetric adjustments in the spine and the lower extremities.

Postural instability resulting from fatigue is the root cause of much bodily inaccuracy and leads to accidents in the cause of prolonged physical activity. Such instability is compensated for in some cases by natural means; thus the body will compensate for deviations of some of its parts from the fundamental standing position. The relation of the line of gravity to the base of support is not affected significantly or consistently when a person assumes different positions of the upper extremities or holds external objects.

Any departure from the balanced posture will strain muscles and ligaments and cause undue friction in joints —if one segment of the body is out of line, all the others will be affected. There appears to be a definite relationship between the alignment of the body segments and the integrity of joints. It is generally accepted that prolonged postural strain is injurious to these structures.

There is adequate clinical evidence that prolonged postural strain is a factor in the arthritic (wearing-out) changes that take place in the weight-bearing joints. It seems certain that the human machine functions more efficiently when the weight-bearing segments are in proper alignment, thus having a minimum of stress and strain on them. When one is sitting, standing or moving about, no undue strain should be put on muscles and joints.

It is probably wrong to assume that there is a common standard of posture for all individuals, even if allowances are made for different body types; neither can we accept one sitting or standing posture as ideal and urge all individuals to aim for it. Certain fundamentals must apply, as has already been stated, but each of us has his own characteristic of educational, occupational, psychological and mechanical influences. The influences of our environment affect mind and body so much that family characteristics are less marked in postures than in such purely inherited traits such as shape of nose and coloring. Postures are to a certain extent attitudes of body and mind, our habitual postures depend largely upon our general health and state of mind. When one is happy and buoyant then one's posture is erect; if one is gloomy then one's posture will be slumped. Since all people are not built alike, there must be a relationship between body-type and posture which is worthy of investigation. The stiff, artificial posture of the soldier standing at attention may look good in a military parade because it makes the men look taller and symbolizes the spirit of aggression, but in ordinary life it is vastly preferable to develop grace.

## 6

# The Importance of Warming-up in Injury Prevention

In the same manner as her professional counterpart on the sports field, the ballet dancer has to "warm up" before commencing strenuous physical activity. It can be justifiably claimed that there is no other factor that has such a vital bearing on the prevention of injuries while dancing. By far the greatest proportion of muscular strains occur because the artiste has gone into her class or her exercises in a "cold" condition. Under such conditions the muscles lack the suppleness that fights off strain and the weakest muscle or group of muscles is damaged by the demands made upon it. A comparison can be made when one considers a motor car, the intelligent owner of which allows the engine to run over on a cold morning, before engaging the gears. He does this because he knows that overnight the oil in the engine has become thickened, and gentle running-in has the effect of lowering the viscosity of the oil by circulating it throughout the engine, thereby warming it and making it liquid. By preliminary exercises, the blood is circulated throughout the body and the muscles become warmed and supple, thus avoiding tearing when put to stress. Body temperature rises in proportion to the intensity of the physical work performed, the higher body temperature furthers the reaction speed of the chemical and physical processes forming the foundation for the greater evolution of energy, which in turn is responsible for greatly increased activity of the body.

An efficient warm-up should accomplish the following things:

> Prepare heart and lungs for hard action so that the discomfort of body adjustments can be eliminated. Get the blood circulating freely throughout the body, moving it from the splanchnic reserve. Ease and release the results of pre-performance or residual tension and construction in key areas. Stretch the key muscles in order to get them ready for fast and effective contraction and to remove any kinks and muscle shortening due to travel, sitting, fatigue carry-over, etc. Make the artist feel loose and ready.

If a proper warm-up procedure is followed out the artist cannot help but be more ready to move efficiently at the beginning of the performance or rehearsal period, be less likely to get hurt, be sharper and physically "up" and be able to endure more efficiently throughout the performance.

Experiments involving track sprinters show that there is a four to six percent improvement in performance by the athlete who has adequately warmed up as opposed to the athlete who has not done so. Improved performances are shown after fifteen minutes preparatory warm-up than when only five minutes is spent on the procedure; warming-up that takes fifteen to thirty minutes shows us marked benefits.

The best results seem to come when no more than five

minutes is allowed to elapse between the conclusion of the warming-up routine and the actual physical activity. Warm clothing, such as tights, leg warmers and a jersey makes the warming-up process more efficient.

It has been suggested that warming-up can be successful when it is carried out by other than actual physical activity. For example, a dancer may be under the misconception that it is adequate to rest in a very hot room, or in a hot bath, immediately prior to her performance. During the course of a series of experiments conducted at the Central Gymnastic Physiological Institute in Stockholm, warming-up by passive means in a steambath was reviewed. It was shown to be appreciably less effective than active warming-up. Improvements in performance over activities without warming-up were slight and cannot compare with actual physical warming-up. All subjects were found to be completely "blown" after a 400 meter run and their degree of exhaustion after activities preceded by steambath warming-up led to the definite conclusion that this method held no advantages.

With well-trained subjects, there is no noteworthy fatigue after fifteen minutes extensive warming-up. So the dancer need not fear that such preliminary activities will produce fatigue during her performance, rather, there will be fatigue PLUS danger if she does NOT carry out a warming-up routine.

Dancers are particularly well placed so far as warming-up procedures are concerned, because much of the warming-up routines are exercises that form an integral part of their training and performance. For instance, a reasonable warming-up procedure might well take the following form:

(1) Stand facing the barre with both hands resting on it.

Two pliés in first position (count one, two three, four).

Four quick grands battements in second position (still facing the barre), R., L., R., L. (count five, six, seven, eight). Repeat three times.

(2) With one hand holding the barre:

Sixteen quick retirés battements, then immediately turn and repeat.

By this time you should feel "all aglow" and ready for your lesson.

The majority of injuries occur for trivial and easily explained reasons, particularly those which take place during teaching. Such a reason is the tiring pupil who is given strenuous exercises toward the end of a training period by a new and fresh teacher. It is obvious that a class will progressively tire as the training goes on, but if more than one teacher is available, the class will be assailed by this fresh instructor, who rarely realizes that her charges are tired while she feels fine. Another cause of injury is in connection with warming-up; if a class is being instructed in some more complicated form of exercise requiring demonstrations, they will thus grow chilled while watching and will eventually enter into the work in a dangerously cold condition. Thus it is essential that dancers are made to warm up more than once during a class, when demonstrations are being given periodically. It is a definite fact that people over thirty years of age are not so supple or resilient as their younger comrades, taking longer to recover from injury and, sometimes fatigue. It is therefore a sensible practice to grade one's training program to allow the older pupil to work in a different fashion to the adolescent or pupil in her early twenties.

Studios and backstage are not always noted for the draft-free warmth; more often than not, they are chill places. It is not only to the dancer's advantage from a performance point of view to adequately warm up; it is also imperative so far as personal freedom from injury is concerned.

7

# Preventing Injury to Children

The importance of ballet training to children is not merely to teach them to dance but to form a basic pattern for their posture and movement throughout their lives. Dancing posture has a definite relationship to everyday posture; inevitably ballet training improves upon the latter. Children will derive from ballet training an enhanced sense of coordination; this is of particular value to boys in later athletic activities. Good posture, fluid movements and a high standard of coordination are all vital factors in fighting off injuries in all forms of sport and physical activity—so the importance of fostering them in children cannot be too highly stressed. It could be claimed that ballet training should be included in every school syllabus, in addition to the Modern Educational Dance and English Country Dancing already covered. Good as they might be, it is possible that these two classes fail in that they do not make the children think quickly enough.

Ballet training does just that: it possesses innumerable facets that have to be thought out. Frequently at the end the pupil has derived a sense of posture, balance, rhythm or movement that will stand her in good stead for the rest of her life. For example, when children first learn they stand with their heels together and knees braced back, "tails" tucked underneath and "tummies" held in; the shoulders are relaxed but pulled down and the head is erect. This is learned through grades six to twelve; then it alters and major work is commenced. Now the pupils find when they do such steps as the PIROUETTE they have to place their weight slightly forward, so they tilt forward from the pelvis. They are unable to maintain a technically correct, upright posture without bending or relaxing the spine. So they allow themselves to bend forward slightly thus giving more balance and control. They have found out something for themselves!

Only a very small proportion of children have the ability or character to become professional dancers. This does not mean that the years of training have been wasted—the physical advantages resulting from ballet training are immense and can have a significant bearing on the child's later life. Ballet schools never get enough children with perfect bodies, natural turn-outs and high extensions. In the best interests of a child, both physically and psychologically, for schools to accept less than those standards is to dangerously expose an unsuitable candidate to arduous and prolonged training. By careful selection and intelligent discrimination by both parent and teacher, the disappointments and the dangers can be avoided.

Ballet training has, perforce, to begin at an early age when it is difficult to predict the growth of the child. At sixteen, the eminently satisfactory shape and proportions possessed at ten years of age may have changed alarmingly!

It is not always possible to tell how a child will develop. She may grow very tall; always a handicap in a dancer or actress as it ties them to certain types of work and restricts their freedom of choice for parts. A ballerina cannot be so tall that few male dancers can partner her. A girl may also get fat and heavy or be markedly underweight and puny so that she finds as she gets older that she is not able to sustain the hard work attached to a dancer's career.

There are certain physical characteristics that are not only aesthetically undeniable but, so far as dancing is concerned, are undersirable handicaps. The short neck and high, or square, shoulders go hand in hand with an upper back and shoulder girdle that is stiff; a tight lower spine and in-turned hips accompany a long back and short thighs. An already arduous schedule is rendered doubly difficult by having such obstacles to surmount. A hollow back with a straight upper spine, often combined with short hamstring muscles and tight lower-back muscles, is most difficult to correct. The slightly sagging posture, indicated by the hollow back and round shoulders of the child who has grown rapidly up to ten years of age, can be straightened up with adequate corrective training.

The naturally good nervous and muscular system possessed by the majority of children greatly aids such correction.

Young children sometimes lack a covering of fat to disguise projecting shoulder blades—a common fault. On the other hand, they can be caused by a contracted chest; this is a condition that requires corrective training, particularly if it is sufficiently far advanced to be classified as a "winged scapula." This should be seen by an orthopedic consultant, just as should any marked asymmetry of the back that makes one shoulder higher than the other or one hip to protrude. While spinal deformities can be caused by faulty habits of standing or by slight and relatively harmless spinal curvatures, they should not be ignored.

This brings up a pertinent point—two, in fact. Orthopedic consultants and their physiotherapists are obviously not always completely in the picture as to what constitutes the basic physical requirements for a dancer. On the other hand, dancing teachers, with their undeniable knowledge and experience of anatomy, capacity, limits and ranges of the human body, should not set themselves up as authorities in those specialized remedial and corrective techniques that lie within the realm of medicine. A little knowledge can sometimes be a dangerous thing; the guiding principle must ALWAYS be that what is being done is in the child's best long-term interests.

The legs are all important; their general shape must be considered together with the size of the thighs and the width of the hips. Wide hips sometimes cause slight knock-knee in girls; this is not abnormal unless—very marked or present in a child of generally frail makeup. In this latter case, they often indicate a general lack of stamina, coupled with poor posture and weak feet. Such signs are often present in children brought up in India or the East. Professional training is too much for these children but their condition can be immensely improved by regular classes. Obvious knock-knees will render their unfortunate owner out for top level dancing, as will bowlegs. The latter are not so important in boys, often accompanying good elevation and sturdy physique. Bowlegs will sometimes straighten as the child grows but tend to leave a flattened, overextended knee that causes a curving backwards of the leg, indicating a weak knee joint with slack ligaments. The majority of conditions respond to treatment, but this one rarely improves and has an adverse effect upon balance, strength and elevation.

A dancer's foot, just as a dancer's body, must never be stiff and tight. A young child's foot must be loose at the ankle joint and the foot itself must possess a low arch. When a foot is stiff, the trouble sometimes lies in the ankle joint above. If a child cannot get a straight line from hip to toe when the foot is pointed (POINTE TENDU in the 4th or 2nd) then look at the ankle joint, which will usually be found to be stiff. Unfortunately, if this is the case at ten years of age, then it will usually be found that the hips and the spine, together with the feet, are equally stiff. This indicates that the child does not have a dancer's body. If a child's foot has a high arch it often spells trouble, because the ligaments of the foot are too long and the muscles weak. The slender, soft flexible foot with long toes seems to go along with delicate hand and long fingers in the same person; it is invariably a weak foot and rarely trains well for ballet.

It is difficult to lay down definite rules about the toes, except to say: beware of the long, overflexible big toe! A long second toe usually behaves itself and often goes with a good, strong reasonably arched foot. Early signs of an enlarged big toe joint must be regarded with suspicion; this is often an inherited tendency. In this connection, children often inherit certain physical characteristics and an initial interview with the parents of a prospective pupil can sometimes be most enlightening!

Having established that any malformation of the body, however slight, calls for special methods suitable to the case, let us consider the child of suitable, normal build. She is a child endowed with the physique of a potential dancer and she is not younger than eight or nine years of age. Tamara Karsavina, famous Russian dancer and Vice-President of the Royal Academy of Dancing until 1955, has written: "It is my firm belief that the strain unavoidable in the strict training of a professional dancer must be spared to the very young. I have watched quite a number of children below the age of eight, coming under the denomination of "child prodigy," to have come to the conclusion that the premature development of muscles arrests the normal growth."

The importance of muscular strength in ballet training cannot be overstressed; the strengthening of the vital muscle groups is the first item on the agenda of professional training. This fact is not always fully appreciated —how often do we find that correct BARRE work is not always followed by the same level of execution in the center? This can only mean one thing—when the support of the BARRE is withdrawn, the strength of the child is insufficient to achieve the EN DEHORS turn while preserving the correct placing. It is interesting to note that the boys at the Bolshoi School in Moscow have their strength, vitality, muscular tone and suppleness developed by a weekly gymnastics class which replaces the Classical Dancing class on Thursdays. The Royal Ballet School now follows this practice, also.

There is a method of strengthening the muscles in a manner specifically suited to ballet training. Dissect any particular exercise into its component parts and practice each part repeatedly until the muscle-group governing the movement is exercised and possesses the desired strength and tension. As an example, take a RONDE DE JAMBE Á TERRE EN DEHORS; an exercise in which the hip frequently turns in before the working foot passes to the first position. Instead of continuous movement, make the pupil hold each of the three main points of the round—DEVANT, EN SECONDE, EN ARRIÈRE, seeing that the thigh is properly tensed. The holding of tension is the way to strengthen the muscle. Perfection of the exercise, once reached, should then be given with a very slight raising of the working foot off the ground. This ensures that the hip muscles are called into action—a good preparation for ADAGE.

BATTEMENTS TENDUS not only develop a properly arched foot but they also strengthen the ankle joint. These are two vital factors because they give to any jump the elasticity upon which depends its quality. Experienced teachers claim, in the first year, to teach up to four sets of BATTEMENTS TENDUS, first to sixteen and later to thirty-two bars of music. In conjunction, DEMI-PLIÉS in all positions, BATTEMENTS TENDUS JETÉS and BATTEMENTS PIQUÉS are given. The same purpose can also be served by RELEVÉ on half-point.* Extension can be developed by concentration on BATTEMENT TENDU JETÉ and GRAND BATTEMENTS. Strength and lightness can be given to the legs and the quality of jumping in length improved by giving up to sixteen by the end of the first year and in the second and third years sixteen in each direction on alternate legs.

A good teacher will not only detect the physical defects of her pupils but she will try to have some idea of the extent to which they can be corrected. She should also be aware of the ways in which this correction can be achieved. Only in this way can children emerge, after two years or so of ballet training, with their faults

* These are not given until later in the syllabus in Great Britain.

corrected, their backs straightened, their turn-out developed, their feet pointed and elevation obtained where it did not previously exist. For example, children with bad turn-out and extension need stretching and limbering exercises done carefully and sparingly; they should only be done after the limbs have been adequately warmed up. A deep cavity, or inner bend in the region of the waist, often accompanied by "winged" shoulder blades, can similarly be corrected by limbering exercises that improve turn-out and extensions at the same time. Specific exercises are to give GRAND PLIÉS lying down, touching the wall in PLIÉ position with the back, behind the bar.

It may be necessary to adapt exercises to compensate for postural deficiencies. For example, knock-knee cannot be corrected and only by adaptation can stability and correct placing of the body be obtained. The student is allowed to slightly incline the body toward the barre, the supporting leg not stretched as fully as normally. In ideal placing, the body is exactly above the legs, on one vertical line, as if an invisible axis went through the very center.

There is a strong case, both physiologically and psychologically, for teaching correct breathing to students. The physical benefits are obvious; the mental factor lies largely in the tension-relieving qualities of correct deep breathing.

Obviously, the wise parent defers to the doctor's judgement so far as her children are concerned, but in the circumstances under discussion this is not enough. Doctors can 'vet' the heart, lungs and general health but they have no knowledge or understanding of those specific stresses and strains imposed upon youthful bodies by ballet training. By experience tempered with instinct, a good teacher can quickly spot physical faults in children, even if she lacks the technical knowledge to give the fault its correct anatomical or pathological label. Clothes hide physical faults; therefore the experienced and wise teacher will insist on giving the child a preliminary physical examination—WITHOUT CLOTHES.

This chapter has merely touched upon the fringes of the many problems connected with the ballet training of children. In the final analysis, much will have to be left to the wisdom and judgement of the teacher in weighing physical attributes against latent talent. Whatever the eventual decision may be, it must ALWAYS be in the best physical interests of the child.

## 8

# Too Fat or Too Lean?

What is the best weight for a dancer? Everyone has a 'best performance' weight, a weight at which she will be at her physical peak and any sudden rise or fall in that weight almost invariably denotes the approach of staleness or lack of training. The weight of the body is Man's visible proof of his organic development; but it must be remembered that two individuals of the same skeletal size may also weigh the same but be vastly different in their respective proportions of muscle, bone and fat. A dancer's weight must, therefore, be considered in terms of the various tissues, allowing that she needs adequate musculature to handle the body weight, plus the bony skeleton, in an efficient fashion.

A moderate amount of adipose tissue is needed for protection against sudden changes of temperature, serving as a cloak to retain the body heat and also as an energy reserve. Too much of this adipose tissue is a sure sign of poor physical condition and, in young people, strength tends to diminish as fat increases. A dancer may be 5 percent overweight and be in a very healthy condition, showing that the body is well nourished and has more than enough of the materials it requires for maintenance and repair. But more than 5 percent is dangerous, proportionate to the percentage she is overweight. To avoid this dangerous condition or to improve their appearance, many people attempt to reduce their overweight, normally using the methods of diet or exercise, or a combination of both.

We are active in our youth, while our bodies are still growing; because of this we do not become overweight. During those same years, an adequate appetite is acquired and digestion is in good shape. At the age of about thirty, when growth has ceased and persons normally become less active, the surplus weight begins to accumulate. A little surplus fat is a healthy condition; it is not wise to be too finely drawn. Reserve energy in the form of fat is stored on the body to resist such emergencies as an illness or injury. While it is sometimes a good thing to have such a surplus, it is important that the life be conducted so as to strike an adequate balance.

People become too fat or too thin—especially too fat —because they do not eat according to their actual physical needs. This is because they have little or no knowledge of how much food they require to provide their bodies with the right amount of fuel for the particular type of life they are living. The average person realizes, in a general sort of way, that a sedentary person, sitting at a desk all day, needs less food than someone who is more active physically. But very few people know how to eat according to their physical needs. If individuals are to sustain their fitness level they must control their weight so that they will not only avoid excess poundage but also get enough fuel to sustain an adequate body weight.

Besides avoiding weight problems, the person who learns how to eat according to her exact needs will also be assured of maximum energy and endurance and will generally eat for maximum protection of her health. To do this, it is necessary for a person to find out her caloric needs per day. This depends upon a number of factors such as age, size, temperament, occupation, time of year, etc. For example, an average man weighing 160 pounds, of average height and normal temperament, working in a sedentary occupation is said to require about 2350 calories per day. The amount of food a person needs to reach her actual daily requirements depends upon the foods and the beverages themselves; some are higher in caloric content than others. Besides eating to one's energy needs, this means that foods and beverages must be chosen according to the nutrients they contain.

There are innumerable books and magazine articles dealing with a person's caloric requirements and outlining the caloric content of certain foods in far greater detail than is possible here; they are worthy of study. It is worth remembering, when dieting, that "fad" diets are usually bad diets!

Foods are fattening only according to their caloric content. The idea that certain foods turn more easily to fat is incorrect. For example, some people think that butter is fattening; although it consists of a large degree of fat, it will not make a person any fatter than any other food containing the same number of calories. Potatoes are a fairly low calory food, the average medium-sized potato contains only about 100 calories, about the same as an ordinary orange. The best practice is to study the caloric content of all the various foods and try to get into the habit of eating those which are low in calories and high in vitamins, minerals and other important nutrients. The only thing that matters at the end of the day, as far as weight is concerned, is the total number of calories that have been eaten.

In cold weather, people burn up more calories because their bodily 'furnace' has to work harder to sustain body heat. A man who works out in the cold is able to take in more calories without getting fat. When a person is on a diet they will lose weight if they stick rigidly to it, regardless of the weather, which doesn't mean that you can eat more in winter! Slightly less sleep than usual will aid in losing weight, because calories are not burned so quickly when one is sleeping. Walking uses calories at the rate of about 110-120 per hour; sleep at 60-70 per hour. The more active one is when reducing the easier and faster will come the results, which is a point in favor of the exercise/diet method advocated later. There is no need to be hungry when on a reducing diet; the great secret of being able to stick with a diet until you have accomplished your objective is to select enough really low calory foods so that your diet has sufficient bulk. This aids in preventing you from feeling hungry, which is the greatest single factor in making people give up dieting.

A person is what they eat, and they must not eat too little of the foods that contain the materials their body requires. At the same time, they must not allow this surplus to become too great so that it becomes a dangerous burden. The first warnings of not eating enough of these essential foods is a feeling of fatigue, lack of energy, listlessness, headaches and spells of dizziness. Many people are so anxious to reduce their weight that they pay little heed to these warnings. A physical breakdown can result.

It is not possible to lose weight without some form of dieting, which causes the body to live on its own surplus. It is a good idea for a person desiring to lose weight to do so by a judicious blending of diet and exercise which enables an ample diet to be consumed without the body being robbed of necessities.

Accepting this, it is easy to see that the dancer is in a particularly advantageous position. The very nature of her activity provides the exercise that will, coupled with the dieting, shed the surplus poundage. This method gives the great dividend of leaving the subject in good physical condition; whereas dieting on its own tends to leave her not only physically weak but muscularly soft.

It has already been stated that a few extra pounds in the young person is not important, children and adolescents being particularly endowed with a youthful chubbiness known as "puppy-fat." This is all very well in the right proportion, but the term "puppy-fat" should not be put forward as an excuse for allowing a child or adolescent to laboriously, and dangerously, carry a stone or so of excess weight around a studio!

Body weight can be increased in a comparatively simple fashioned; however, the value of the resulting increase is not of any importance unless the gain is useable weight in the form of muscle bulk. Most people embarking upon a weight-increasing program merely add superfluous fat which actually cuts down on their efficiency rather than increasing it. Unless the increase is in the form of muscle bulk, a dancer will merely exchange a loss of agility, timing, endurance and stamina for the added weight. Remember, even four or five pounds of excess fat has a detrimental effect upon a person's mechanical skill, energy and endurance.

If you have no special reason for increasing your weight then you are best off lean—unless, of course, you are markedly underweight. Some dancers want to put on weight for aesthetic reasons—they feel that they would look better. Others believe that they would like to fill in a few hollows and round out some angles because this will be an indication of good health and fitness.

The dancer who is obviously underweight for her age and height should only take remedial steps under the guidance of her doctor. There is often a physical reason demanding proper medical supervision. An individual's body weight is largely dependent upon body type, temperament and the life she leads. This indicates that it is possible, in trying to add body weight, to destroy some natural skills and talents in exchange for added pounds.

There are two ways in which body bulk can be increased—one is exercise, the other is diet. The former may well be outside the scope of the young dancer, both for the reasons of strength and because the type of exercise might well have a detrimental effect upon her dancing. The only effective exercise method is by supervised body building using weights.

The diet schedule will require you to eat more calories per day than you actually require. To find out your daily calorific requirements to increase weight—multiply your present weight (in pounds) by twenty, then add 3,000 calories per day. The foods you eat must be high in calories and full of the necessary nutrients; particularly important are protein foods because of the role they play in building, repairing and sustaining body tissues. The list will include: cashew nuts, figs, honey, ice cream, cream, whole milk, cheese, whole-grain breads and cereals, butter, creamed soups, custards, beans, potatoes. Eat plenty of meat and fresh fruit and vegetables; although not particularly high in calories, they are packed full of necessary vitamins and minerals.

A drink, known as a "Block-buster" taken by the tumbleful between meals will really give results; it consists of 20 percent cream, two teaspoonfuls of honey and the juice of four oranges.

When a person wants to eat heavily, an appetite problem can arise—you just don't feel like shoveling down all this food! Ask your doctor for an appetite-improving tonic; Vitamin B-12 is a good one.

The dancer will find, by the very nature of her activities, that it is difficult to add weight. The less active a person is then the easier it will be for them to increase their weight. A person on a weight-gaining schedule should have a minimum of ten hours sleep per night and a twenty minutes rest after each meal. A big effort should be made to relax, to slow down on mental and emotional activity and to avoid fussing and worrying.

Because of body type and temperament, some people will find it easier than others to increase their muscle bulk. Under thirty years of age, if not medically underweight, try to remain as lean as possible, although when you are young a few extra pounds are not serious. Over thirty, the leaner you are, the healthier you will be; you will feel fitter and live longer.

Allowing that there is a certain degree of importance in both slimming and weight-gaining, it must be remembered that the human body is a very delicate, intricate and balanced mechanism. Any sort of program or way of life, which affects it must be intelligently planned and supervised or harm, rather than good, can result.

# 9

# The Teacher's Role when Injuries Occur

The prime role of the teacher is to teach dancing and not to treat injuries—as in so many spheres of modern life, time is the guiding factor. The teacher must have sufficient personality and character to instill into her pupils the importance of "self-treatment" so that they cheerfully carry out at home the often monotonous remedial exercises that she has shown them.

Most teachers are conscious that they are expected to be walking encyclopedias on the various ailments and injuries liable to affect their pupils. This takes the form of being asked complex questions on diet, fatigue, cramp, stitch, etc., etc. This book will cope with many of these queries and commonsense will fill the gaps. A very useful foundation on which to build is to undertake a first aid course under the auspices of the Red Cross. Here will be learned the vital maxim: "When in doubt, send for a doctor."

Every studio should have a first aid box that is readily accessible. A kit containing the following items will enable anything but a really serious injury to be tackled competently.

*Treatment of wounds*

Solution of mild Dettol, use in cleansing the wounds.

Acriflavine in saline, for dressing small grazes, etc.

Acriflavine emulsion, for dressing larger wounds that require covering.

Collodion, a "liquid skin" solution, painted on.

Adrenalin, aids in controlling bleeding, applied on a pad.

*Treatment of bruises*

Lead and opium lotion, used as a soothing dressing for bruises

Liniment A. B. C. (aconite, belladonna and chloroform) applied to a bruise as a counter-irritant (highly poisonous).

Chili paste (capiscum vaseline) massaged into a bruised area will bring warmth and relief from pain.

*Dressings*

3 in. wide rolls of elastoplast (or similar adhesive elastic bandages).

1 in. and 2 in. rolls of zinc oxide plaster.

Adhesive strip dressing.

$2\frac{1}{2}$ in. cotton bandages.

3 in. crepe bandages.

Triangular bandages.

Cotton wool.

Roll of gauze.

Roll of lint.

Safety pins.

*General*

Friar's balsam (tincture benzoin) used before applying adhesive plaster, also may be used as an inhalant.

Ether or methylated spirit used to clean skin and remove plaster.

Talcum powder, used for toilet purposes or for massage.

Sal volatile, used in cases of faintness.

Codeine or aspirin, relieves pain and minor malaise.

Calamine lotion, relieves skin irritation and sunburn.

Vaseline, prevents chafing of limbs, stops dressing sticking.

Smelling salts, aid in reviving after faintness or loss of consciousness.

Scissors.

Small bowl.

Eye lotion and eye bath.

Razor for shaving limbs before applying plaster.

Forceps or tweezers, used in dressing where gauze etc., is not to be touched by hand.

Massage oil.

Towel and soap.

The type of conditions that might require initial treatment in the studio are:

> Contusions
> Lacerations
> Abrasions
> Sprains
> Strains
> Fractures and dislocations
> Cramp
> Concussion
> Eye injuries (foreign body in eye).

The immediate treatment for these conditions is described in the respective chapters. It may be necessary to suggest that heat be applied to an injured part; some homes possess an infra-red lamp or an electric "bowl-fire" that can be used for this purpose. But, a very simple and easily applied form of heat can be given by means of "contrast-baths"—the alternate bathing of the injured part in hot and cold water. Another similar and equally effective treatment is that of hot towels; a folded towel is wrapped around the injured part and hot water poured continually over it. Both of these forms of heat have an extremely soothing and relaxing effect. Hot water bottles are also useful but in all cases every precaution should be taken to ensure that burns are not caused by overenthusiasm.

A teacher must ensure that no dancer returns to practice or actual performances without being 100 percent fit for the work in question. It is not an easy matter to handle, as dancers are invariably enthusiastic people and will often claim to be completely free from pain and limitation of movement solely in order that they may speedily return to their beloved dancing. On the other hand, there is a minority who will, for some purpose of their own (either conscious or subconscious), claim to be far worse than they really are. They will linger on, having treatment long after the injury has little more left than nuisance value.

Even in the world of professional sport there is little system used in determining whether an athlete is fit to resume playing. As in the world behind the footlights, nothing more scientific than common sense is used when testing an athlete recently recovered from injury. This must mean that there is always the risk of the performer breaking down in public or working under conditions of pain and difficulty. It is possible however to evolve a simple routine that not only prevents a breakdown but also enhances the teacher's reputation! Consider the following points, in the order given:

1. *Appearance*—Contrast the injured part with the un-injured limb, look for swelling, redness, fluid, un-even contours, breaks in the skin.

2. *Everyday Function*—Before the patient is actually tested observe her normal movements, watch for a limp, notice how she ascends and descends stairs if possible, and how she sits and rises from a chair. It is often possible to detect a guarded movement, or a "carrying" of the injured part, as the pupil is not conscious that she is being observed and subsequently is not braced up to give the impression of fitness.

3. *Questioning*—By means of clear-cut questions and answers it is often possible to ascertain a person's degree of physical fitness. Few people will answer "Yes" to an outright question: "Are you fit enough to dance properly?" if there remains a doubt in their own mind.

4. *Pain*—On movement, and on pressure. It is often found that an injured part will remain tender to pressure of the fingers long after the pupil is fit enough to dance, but pain on movement persisting after the pupil has "warmed up" denotes that a dangerous degree of injury still persists.

5. *Passive Movements*—Tell the patient to remain completely limp and put all the muscles around the injury to their fullest degree of stretching. Pain denotes that some degree of injury remains.

6. *Active Movements*—Tell the patient to move the injured part while the teacher applies some mild resistance to the movement. It is possible in this fashion to test all the muscle groups, both prime movers and antagonists, thus speedily ascertaining if an injured area remains.

7. *Resistance Exercises*—Before an athlete or dancer can be considered 100 percent fit the joint or muscle that has been injured must be brought to a point where it is actually fitter than the uninjured counterpart on the opposite side of the body. As an example, if the knee joint received an injury the main principle of treatment would be to maintain the strength and "tone" of the quadriceps muscles of the thigh. By means of attaching weights to the feet it is possible to test that muscle group when sitting with the legs dangling over the edge of a couch or table, and alternately extending and flexing the knee. The uninjured leg should be tested first and a note taken of the maximum amount of weight that it is capable of lifting ten times in succession. The injured leg is then tested similarly, and should not be considered fit until it can lift at least as much, but preferably more weight than the other leg. The reason for this test is that obviously the injured leg has to compensate for the period of disability and resulting weakness, consequently it needs more power to do this.

8. *Functional Tests*—The pupil should be put through a very thorough test in the studio or rehearsal room. After a more-than-thorough warming-up period, the pupil should be put through a strenuous routine—at first "flowing" and then performing sudden, almost "jerky" movements. There are movements outside those of dancing which may be utilized such as short sprints and running a small "figure-of-eight" course, turning rapidly on word of command, swerving, jumping etc. Any signs of pain or limitation of movement rule the pupil out. It is far better to break down during a test rather than an actual performance.

The teacher has to be something of a psychologist when dealing with dancers, who are frequently high strung and of a temperamental nature. This means that they must always be treated as individuals, given sympathy when necessary and firmness when the occasion demands. It is sometimes necessary to "kid" performers to obtain the best out of them; the implied faith and confidence in their ability giving them the assurance they lack so that they can produce their best efforts when required.

Today's standards are so high that the difference between one dancer and another is often as much a matter of morale as of technical ability. In the leading ballet companies, all the dancers are of a very high technical standard and may differ only slightly in their potentials. This means that frequently the dancer keyed to the highest pitch is the most successful. From these remarks it can be seen that it is very useful for a teacher to have some idea of psychology when dealing with dancers because their preparation is partly a problem of mental conditioning.

Self-confidence is an essential part of every dancer's make-up; it is the factor that makes for success. The teacher should never delude a pupil into thinking that she is perfect; but should honestly assess the pupil's capabilities and then add 25 percent for good measure. Every dancer approaches a performance in a nervous condition, but if she can add confidence to her ability and training background, then she has got away to a flying start.

# PART III
# VITAL AREAS OF THE BODY

# 10

# The Foot—It's Structure and Hygiene

Ever since Man became erect and ceased to walk on all fours he has been having trouble with his feet, which are among the most vulnerable parts of the body. To the conditions of painful feet, sweating feet, swollen feet, and odorous feet can now be added the sportsman's own condition—athlete's foot. While great attention is given to the rest of the body, the feet are frequently neglected; if the hand is hurt it can be put into a sling but no such facilities exist for the feet.

The feet suffer constant minor injuries and irritations; unfortunately one pair of feet has to last a lifetime. The foot acts as a springy organ of locomotion to prevent jars to the brain, spinal cord, and abdominal and pelvic organs. In a "highly tuned" individual such as a ballet dancer, general health can often be in direct ratio to the condition of her feet; foot injuries can cause adverse reactions in the leg, knee, hip, back and spine.

The foot consists of twenty-six bones, in three distinct groups; the tarsus, metatarsus and the phalanges. The tarsus is formed of seven bones; the talus, calcaneus, navicular, cuboid and the 1st, 2nd and 3rd cuneiform bones. There are five metatarsal bones and fourteen phalanges.

So that the foot can support the body weight in an

erect posture with the least expenditure of material, it is constructed of a series of arches formed by the tarsal and metatarsal bones, strengthened by the ligaments and tendons of the foot. The main arches are the internal (medial) arch, the external (lateral) arch, and the transverse arch. The Medial arch is formed by the calcaneus, talus, navicular, the three cuneiform bones and the 1st, 2nd and 3rd metatarsal bones. The summit of the arch is the uppermost surface of the talus, and the piers on which it rests in standing are the tuberosity of the calcaneus at the rear and the 1st, 2nd and 3rd metatarsals in the front. Its characteristics are a high degree of elasticity due to the height of the arch and to the number of small joints between its component parts. The weakest part is the joint between the talus and the navicular, which is braced by a strong structure known as the spring ligament; it is also strengthened internally by blending with the deltoid ligament of the ankle joint, and is supported underneath by the fan-shaped insertion of the tibialis posticus muscle. The arch is further supported by the plantar fascia, the small muscles in the sole of the foot, the tendons of the tibialis anticus and posticus muscles and of the peroneus longus muscle, and also by the ligaments of all small joints that are involved in the structure of the arch.

The Lateral arch is formed by the calcaneus, cuboid and the 4th and 5th metatarsals. Its chief joint is that between the calcaneus and the cuboid, and possesses a special locking mechanism which allows only limited movement. The most marked features of this arch are its solidarity and its small elevation. It has two strong ligaments, the long plantar and the calcaneo-cuboid ligaments, which in conjunction with the tendons of the extensor muscles and the short muscles of the little toe, do much to support this arch.

The Transverse arch forms a complete dome in the middle of the foot when both feet are placed alongside each other. It is strengthened by the interrosseus muscles which run lengthways between the metatarsal bones, and by the plantar and dorsal ligaments, by the short muscles to the fifth toe and by the tendon of the peroneus longus muscle, which stretches across the foot between the piers of the arches.

It should be constantly borne in mind that a dancer can miss a vital performance through an infected blister or an ingrowing toe nail just as easily as by a strained muscle or joint. Just as in Life, one only gets as much back as one puts in, so a foot will respond to demands made upon it in direct proportion to the amount of care it is given. A dancer should maintain a high standard of general foot hygiene and possess an elementary knowledge of the essentials of chiropody. There is much in the treatment of simple foot conditions that can come under the heading of plain common sense; the prevention of blisters, hard and soft corns, hard skin and ingrowing toenails is not beyond the scope of the individual.

The healthy foot must be clean; it must frequently be washed with warm water and soap, and if the foot requires hardening then cold water should be used. Never soak the feet in water, as this softens them, allows blisters to form and aggravates sweating. After washing, the feet must be thoroughly dried, particularly between the toes where the soft, thin skin quickly becomes sore and tender if inadequate or incorrect drying is performed, thus causing soft corns.

The correct routine for foot hygiene is as follows:

The shoes must be dry and clean, the socks must be frequently washed, rubbed soft and carefully darned, if required. Wash the feet in warm (or cold, if preferred) water, thoroughly dry, rub with methylated spirits. Correctly treat blisters, corns and abrasions, and finally use a foot powder, put on clean socks and light shoes. A cheap and very good foot powder can be made from 10 parts of boric acid powder, 3 parts of salicylic acid and 87 parts of powdered talc.

A big factor in the care of the feet is the type and the condition of the shoes and socks, which must always be of the correct size and fitting. Shoes or socks that are too tight across the toes cause a distortion of the foot known as hallux valgus, in which the big toe is forced outwards and presses against the second toe thus causing a bunion of the projecting head of the metatarsal bone a little down the foot. Socks must be watched for shrinkage, frequent and careful washing will keep them soft and pliable, besides greatly prolonging their lives, as normal sweat of the foot is absorbed into the sock and will tend to rot it, besides affecting the skin.

The children should be encouraged to wear cotton or woollen socks for class in preference to nylon. In the same way wool tights are preferable for practice—though of course, not so glamorous!!

Blisters are caused by friction and irritation; they are prevented by soaping the feet to lessen the friction, hardening the feet by the use of spirit, alum powder in the socks or bathing in alum water. A thrice-weekly bathing in a one percent solution of formalin will harden the feet very adequately. When a blister has occurred the treatment must be carried out under conditions of the utmost sterility: needles used to prick the blister must have been boiled or held in flame, and after the blister has been painted with iodine or acriflavine, then a dry dressing is applied.

The nails must be cleaned along their free edge, and sides, where dirt and dead skin gather. This is important, otherwise an infection of the nail-bed will follow if the skin is broken. Cut the nails straight across. Failure to do this results in that painful condition known as ingrowing toenails, in which the nail border presses into the nail fold instead of merely resting on it, eventually growing into the nail fold. The patient usually aggravates the condition by cutting off the offending corner, so that when the toe bears weight the skin in front of the nail edge tends to fold over it, causing the nail to press against the skin as it grows forward. The treatment is to remove the inflammation by bathing the foot or toe in hot water, or by applying hot fomentations. Gently press a flattened tinfoil guard or a piece of cotton wool under the projecting piece of nail, thus protecting the tender skin beneath nail, and guiding the nail as it grows forward out of the little hole in which it has become buried. A means of alleviating a minor ingrowing nail is to file a groove down the center of the nail, thus allowing the nail to buckle slightly in the middle and take pressure off its edges.

Corns and callosities are painful but unfortunately common. The corns can be hard or soft, and are due to mechanical irritation such as an illfitting shoe. The outer horny layer of the skin is stimulated to overgrowth, especially in the center of the irritated area, and this presses downward on the deeper skin, which is sensitive —hence pain results. Callosities are due to local mechanical irritation also, such as the constant use of a tool or a golf club bearing on the same portion of the fingers or the palm of the hand. The prevention of corns and callosities is obviously to take pressure off the sensitive part, by mean of correctly fitting shoes, etc. The treatment of this condition is to paint salicylic acid on the offending area for a few days, causing a softening which will allow a paring away with correctly sterilized chiropody tools. Prevent pressure by means of pads of sponge rubber or adhesive felt cut in a lifebuoy fashion with the hole over the sensitive part. Soft corns between the toes can be treated by means of cotton-wool impregnated with foot powder, changed daily.

Know your limitations. Do not worsen a condition by trying to save the cost of a visit to a chiropodist. The regular services of a good, experienced and adequately qualified chiropodist is money well spent.

One does not have to be an athlete to suffer from "Athlete's Foot," a troublesome, highly contagious condition peculiar to Man; it is caused by a fungus, Epidermophyton Inguinale. The lesions are first noticed in the cleft of the little toe; they take the form of small blisters often on a reddish ground. They may also be in common form of dead white skin, made soft by the prevailing moist condition of the toe cleft. The treatment consists of daily painting with Castellani's paint or gentian violet; another firm favorite is Whitfield's ointment.

A similar condition is known as Dhobi's itch, an infection found in the groin and invariably caused by the infection of athlete's foot being carried to that area, sometimes weeping and painfully irritating. It is obvious that if one wishes to remain free from Dhobi's itch one should not catch the primary condition, Athlete's foot; otherwise the daily application of 3.5 percent iodine will clear it up.

# 11

# Common Foot Injuries Incurred by Dancers

There is no member of the community to whom the feet are more important than to the dancer; it is from the feet upwards that the whole silhouette is built. They are the basic foundation of an artist's performance so that weak and unstable feet will permit only a weak and unstable performance. The feet of a dancer must be strong, flexible and sensitive, possess character and be as expressive in movement as the hands and face, plus being muscularly developed to bear the weight of the body. This requires a perfect formation of bone and muscle achieved by years of hard work; a dancer should bestow individual care upon her feet from the moment she begins her side practice.

A dancer should be taught to place her feet correctly on the ground and not to "turn out" more than her hips will allow: to be well "turned out" is a necessity to every dancer. It is far from easy for the body weight to be correctly and adequately transmitted to feet which are turned out at 180°; this is particularly the case when jumping. In her eagerness to do well, a dancer will often try to "turn out" from the ankles by allowing her feet to roll in, as shown in Figs. 1 and 2. In this way, flat

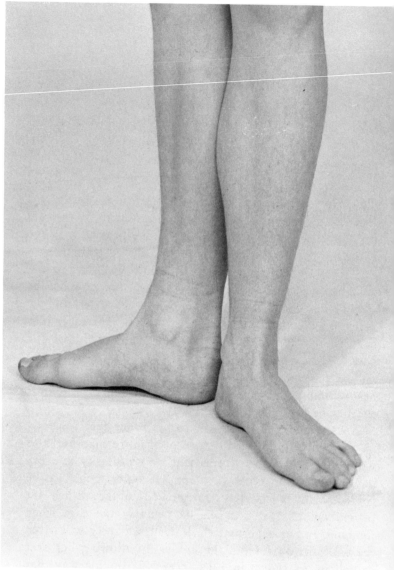

Fig. 1. Correct

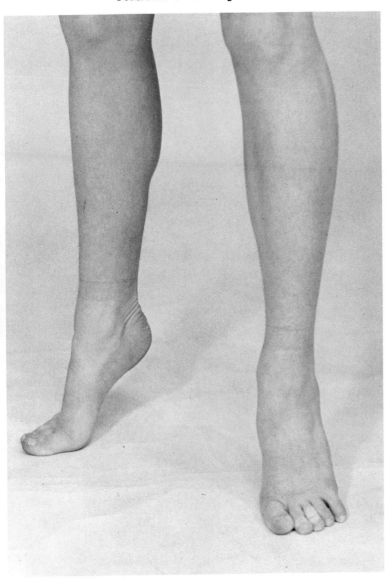

Fig. 2. Incorrect

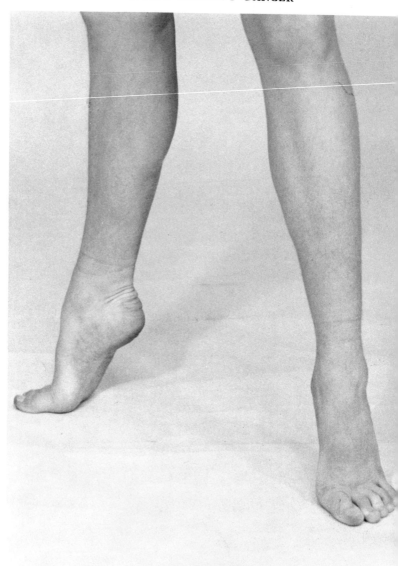

Fig. 3. Correct

foot is caused by the dropping of the instep, together with strain of associated tendons; inflamed toe joints can also result.

If, in an attempt to avoid rolling, the foot is turned so that the big toe is lifted, (Figs. 3 and 4) other injuries can be caused. The underneath surfaces of the heads of the metatarsal bones can be bruised or the tranverse arch at the front of the foot can be strained. This position can also cause a "stress" (or "march") fracture of one of the shafts of the 2nd, 3rd or 4th metatarsal bones. Its onset is sudden and initially indicated by pain running through the foot, with tenderness to finger-pressure on both top and bottom surfaces of the foot. A stress fracture is not usually detectable by x-ray in its early stages but becomes more obvious as bony repair takes place; local tenderness, and pain on jumping can be felt for three weeks or so. It is necessary to immobilize the foot in a walking plaster or to firmly bind it in elastoplast. This is a job for the doctor or hospital.

By developing the small (intrinsic) muscles of the foot so that the outer toes grip the floor and support the foot arches without the big toe joint being lifted, weight can be properly transmitted to that joint with no flattening of the arches. (See Figs. 5 and 6).

The toes must all be on the ground; the arch well lifted—it should be possible to insert the fingers underneath it—and the body weight toward the outside of the foot. When rising onto the Demi-Pointe, work from the heel right through the middle of the foot on to the Demi-Pointe. Make sure it is the Demi-Pointe and NOT the ball of the foot! The line of the leg should be straight from the metatarsal arch, and the body balanced on the length of the toes.

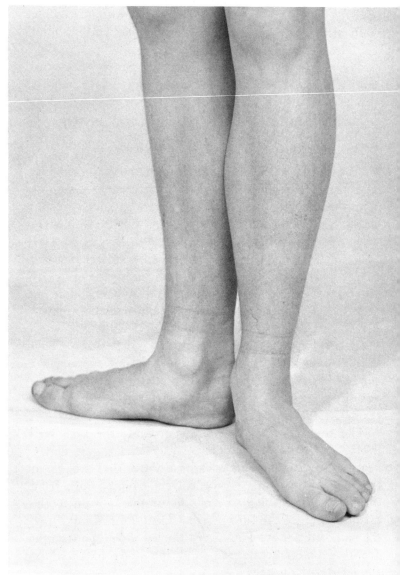

Fig. 4. Incorrect

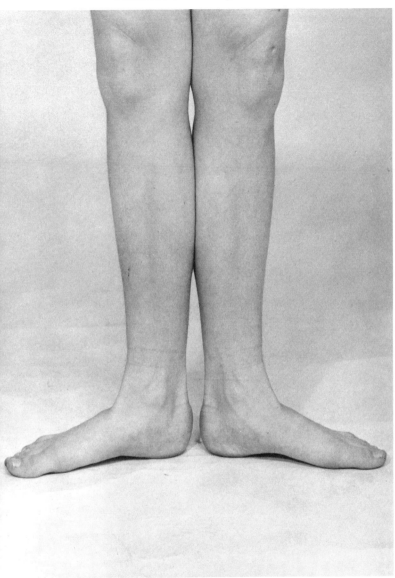

Fig. 5.

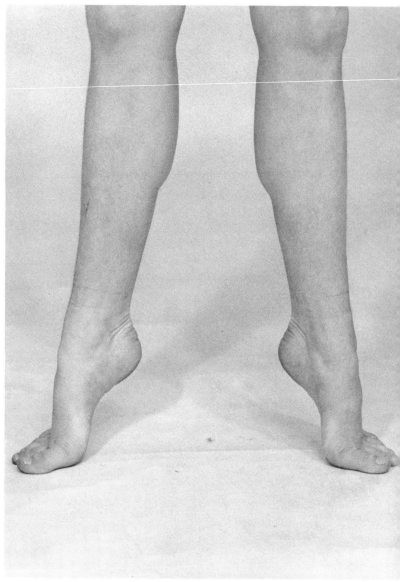

Fig. **6.**

The dancer should learn how her feet and legs work. Let her hold her leg quite straight in front of her with the foot turned up from the ankle as far as possible, then slowly—through the center of the foot—push the foot down until the instep is fully stretched, taking care that the ankle is in the correct position, the heel directly underneath, the toes straight and not curled. Having achieved this correctly, then turn the leg out from the hip, maintaining the position of foot, whether Devant, Derrière or De Côté.

The foot should never be permitted to stray in the opposite direction, so that the inside ankle joint protrudes and the weight is thrown entirely on the big toe; this can result in an enlarged, inflamed and painful joint.

The big toe joint is most important to a dancer and should receive adequate respect. For instance, when a big toe is disproportionately long it is liable to bend inwards in Pointe work; this tends to enlarge or even dislocate its joint. To prevent this, the shoes worn for Pointe work should be reinforced by a strip of leather glued inside; the strip must fill the space under the arch and, if required, can be extended to give support to the big toe joint. Another precautionary measure to avoid injuring the joint is to have a pad of cotton wool between the big and the second toe; or a specially devised orthopedic appliance can be utilized. The dancer who has a big toe that is longer than the second toe needs to be particularly careful as it can lead to Hallux Valgus. This is a condition in which the big toe is forced or deflected outwards, sometimes becoming so marked that it is displaced behind the second toe. If the top of the big toe is inclined toward the little toe, then the lower end of the big toe is forced in the opposite direction, causing a prominence on the inside of the foot. Inevitably with the passing of time, on this bulge a bunion forms; pain and discomfort arise from this inflamed area and are made worse by footwear and Pointe work. Hallux Valgus can also cause a splaying of the forefoot with consequent stretching of the ligaments and an abnormal distribution of weight onto the heads of the outer few metatarsal bones; all these factors giving rise to pain and discomfort.

In early cases of Hallux Valgus, the treatment should be directed at removing the cause; thus correct footwear must be worn and dancing shoes padded to prevent friction. It is important to check that footwear, both outdoor and stage, is big enough. The tendency toward splaying of the forefoot should be counteracted by exercises of a remedial nature designed to strengthen the muscles of the sole of the foot and the calf. If this is not sufficient, a metatarsal pad of felt or sponge rubber can be fitted to the sole of the foot and worn with outdoor shoes. (It is doubtful whether such an appliance could be worn with dancing shoes). Such a pad supports the heads of the 2nd, 3rd and 4th metatarsals and prevents splaying of the foot.

In more advanced cases, operative treatment is necessary in which the prominence on the inside of the foot is surgically chiseled off. If arthritis has developed in the joint, the joint is surgically re-modelled (Keller's Operation) and the arthritic excrescences removed. After-treatment consists of moving the joint as soon as the stitches are removed; emphasis being given to abduction of the toe (inward movement toward the center line of the body).

Male dancers mostly wear soft and tightly fitting

dancing shoes; they cause continual mild irritation to the big toe joint. This leads to a condition known as Hallux Rigidus, in which enlargement of the joint causes limitation of the normal range of movement of the big toe. At first, this is confined to increasing inability to raise the toe upwards, but time causes the remaining movements to be affected until ultimately a completely stiff joint results. The active nature of a dancer's foot movements may cause excessive mobility in adjoining joints in an attempt to compensate, leading to a dislocation. Obviously, Hallux Rigidus is a serious problem that will affect a dancer's ability to jump. There is a pain and swelling in the joint, particularly in adolescents; the pain is most marked when walking and becomes worse when dancing.

In many cases, Hallux Rigidus is associated with other weaknesses of the foot leading to greater liability of the big toe joint to injury. Adolescents with long narrow feet which are inclined to turn out when weight-bearing are particularly subject to this condition as weight is then borne on the inner aspect of the joint. This gives rise to inflammation and subsequent limitation of movement. In the adult the condition is associated with bad shoes; constant stubbing of the big toe is a common cause. The trouble never spreads to other joints.

When considering the adolescent it is well to look out for early inflammation in this joint and to institute remedial measures. Where no bony changes are present, the condition is best treated in its acute stage by immobilization in plaster. Later, attention should be directed to restore, by remedial exercises, the tone of the small muscles of the foot, correct weight-bearing should be encouraged and suitable shoes worn.

The generally accepted forms of treatment are not easy to carry out when dealing with dancers, consisting as they do of the provision of a rocker sole to the patient's shoe, so that she pivots instead of extending her big toe. The other accepted alternative seems to be a metatarsal bar put straight across the sole at the metatarsal heads.

Early Hallux Rigidus can be treated at home by the sufferer: twice or thrice daily bathe the foot in alternative hot and cold water ("Contrast baths"). The hot water should be as hot as can be comfortably borne and all possible toe movements carried out in it; the cold water is to provide the contrast. On completion of the contrast bathing, gently manipulate the toe; bending movements should be accompanied by "traction," a stretching forward of the toe in an effort to separate the joint surfaces. For walking and exercise, fix on the underneath of the toe a support of felt stiffened by adhesive plaster.

Often, a patient will "flare-up" a mild, prevalent condition of Hallux Rigidus and treatment will usually be required for three or four days. Such a procedure may occur three or four times a year. Manipulation by a trained physiotherapist, followed by mobilizing exercises, is also a very useful method of treatment. When the condition is severe and osteo-arthritic changes have occurred, surgical operation becomes necessary. Again, Keller's Operation is performed and the results are highly successful although the dancer must be prepared for three or four months away from full dancing activity.

The forefoot is constructed to bear only about one-third of the body weight; when an excessive proportion of the body weight falls upon it, such as when the toes are taking none of this weight, then pain is caused on the under surface of the foot, just below the toes. It is a condition caused by strain, toxic influences (See Chapter 20.) or any factor which results in loss of tone of muscles of the feet. These causes produce a tenderness in the under part of the capsules of the middle three metarso-phalangeal joints. The pain is situated beneath the heads of the metatarsals (just below the toes) ; it is continuous and burning. It can sometimes cause actual wasting of the small muscles of the feet; coupled with typical exquisite tenderness this inevitably leads to alteration in posture and muscular imbalance—both vital to the dancer.

Metatarsalgia is produced when a dancer jumps and lands heavily on an uneven, rough surface, or onto a pebble or similar small object, or through incessant jumping-and-landing. It can be secondary to another condition such as an ankle sprain, when excessive and unaccustomed strain is placed upon the foot. Or it can be postural and associated with the same factors that cause painful flat foot. Metatarsalgia can follow a rest period or an illness, when the flexor muscles of the toes become weak so that insufficient weight is borne by the pads of the toes. This means that excessive pressure is placed upon the metatarsal heads.

Early treatment of metatarsalgia consists of taking weight-bearing pressure off the metatarsal heads by means of suitably shaped pads of sponge rubber on the under surface of the foot. Elastoplast strapping around the foot also helps normal walking. Exercises should also be given to strengthen flexor muscles of the toes, such as flexing them against resistance; standing on tiptoe, heels raising and lowering and by picking up marbles and pencils etc. with the toes. By enabling the toes to strongly flex during weight-bearing, they will bear more weight and take painful pressure off the metatarsal heads.

When home treatment fails to relieve the intense tenderness, it will be necessary to have physiotherapy; this consists of shortwave diathermy heat, deep-friction massage, electrical stimulation of foot muscles and exercises.

Extending from the calcaneum bone (the heel) to the four outer toes is a sheet of pure fibrous tissue known as the plantar fascia, damage to which causes extreme pain, limitation of movement, and, sometimes, deformity. It is subject to strain and sprain in all jarring movements such as leaping or jumping, and, in cases of flatfoot, is under considerable tension. Damage to the plantar fascia will most often manifest itself in the form of a dull, bruised feeling, particularly on pressure whether by the exploratory fingers or when walking. It is a troublesome condition to clear up, being prolonged and obstinate; the deep heating obtained from short wave diathermy is about the only means of getting at it, other than by almost complete rest, with nonweight-bearing foot exercises and quadriceps exercises. Protection in the form of adhesive felt pads or shaped pieces of sponge rubber will frequently enable the sufferer to continue working after the condition has passed the acute stage. Deep manipulations with the fingertips (in the form of massage) will increase the local blood supply and aid in dispersing the accumlated products of bruising.

Obviously, there is not a great deal of superficial tissue on the bones forming the upper surface of the foot, consequently a kick or knock will cause extreme pain and will remain a painful area for a long time. The application of cold compresses or evaporating lotions immediately after the injury is sustained, followed by contrast baths, or by heat and massage on the following day, will clear up the condition eventually, while foot exercises must be carried out during the period of incapacity or for as long as the pain causes the dancer to walk in a guarded fashion. It will frequently be found that the patient will have pain and weakness in the ligaments of the sole of the foot following ankle sprains, and foot exercises and contrast baths should be carried out when this is the case.

# 12

# Strengthening the Small Muscles of the Foot

Foot ache is a warning, pain is a danger signal and swelling can be dangerous, so adequate care must be taken of these signs. Foot fatigue is treated by means of rest, bathing with alternate hot and cold water, temporary application of supporting padding or strapping. Chronic foot fatigue is often caused by muscular weakness, when the "intrinsic" or small muscles of the soles of the feet are failing to do their work. These muscles are mainly responsible for keeping the bones of the foot in such a position as to maintain the arches and to permit trouble-free movement of the foot.

The causes of chronic foot fatigue are continued neglect, associated injury, the after-effects of illness, and incorrectly fitting shoes and socks. Through one or more of these reasons the muscles lose some of their tone and strength, allowing the bones over which they run, and to which they are attached, to fall into incorrect positions permitting strain and stress to fall upon the ligaments, which are inelastic structures ill-constructed to bear such strains. To commence wearing arch supports and the like is to condemn the feet to suffer permanently from this condition; the sole cure is to reeducate the muscles concerned so that they will once again competently carry out their task.

The only known method of reeducating muscle is by exercise and the feet are no exception, but in the case of the feet the principal aim must be to mobilize the foot before strengthening it. This is done by light, rhythmic-type exercises, consisting of flexion and extension of the toes, and of the metatarsal/tarsal joints and by self-manipulation. This is done by sitting with one leg crossed over the other, the offending foot grasped firmly with one hand while the other hand limits the movement to the joints required by holding the rear portion of the foot. All possible movements are passively carried out, stretching, flexing, extending, rotating the toes and joints, until the foot is supple and ready for strengthening exercises. These may be made into amusing sessions, consisting as they do of such items as picking up pencils, marbles and small coins with the toes, by placing a duster with its point under the toes and, by means of "scrabbling" movements, drawing the entire duster under the foot, by so parting all the toes as to see daylight between each pair—by no means an easy task. An extremely good exercise of a more conventional nature is called "foot shortening" and consists of raising the inner arch of the foot by pressing the pads under the tips of the toes down onto the ground. Without actually flexing them, hold the arch-raising position for a few seconds, relax and continue. All these exercises should be incorporated in a thrice-daily routine, or more if possible.

A painful, bruised feeling persistently irritating the sole of the foot is often caused by landing on a hard surface. When landing after a jump, this bruised feeling is often experienced by a person with some degree of flat foot. This extreme pain and limitation of movement is caused by inflammation or bruising of the plantar fascia, a sheet of fibrous tissue extending beneath the skin from the heel to the toes on the sole of the foot. It is an obstinate and troublesome condition difficult to clear up. Pressure must be taken off the tender area by means of pads of sponge rubber or felt, and daily sessions of deep friction-type massage with the finger tips will aid. The only known form of heat which will affect this condition is short wave diathermy, on account of its deep-lying position.

Before the condition of the feet becomes as far advanced as the cases already considered, there are ways in which the dancer can tone up and revitalize her feet. They are methods which should help to give the suppleness and flexibility in the coordinated use of the feet that will make the execution of the difficult "PAS" easier and technically more brilliant.

Whenever possible, practice BATTERIE lying on the back, on the floor, thus taking the weight of the body off the feet. ENTRECHATS and CHANGEMENTS can be very advantageously practiced in this position. Raise the legs, hold them vertically so that the toes point to the ceiling; practice the movements slowly, quickening as they become more fluent. Still in this position, stretch the toes straight up to the ceiling and then bend them back from the ankle so that the toes point towards the head. This movement can also be taken sitting up quite straight with the legs stretched out in front, the toes still stretched up to the ceiling. This also stretches the tendons at the back of the knees and strengthens the muscles of the legs.

Press the toes forward and up again; then divide the

feet, keeping the heels together; with them still braced, push one foot over to the right and one foot over to the left. This flexes the ankles and braces the instep.

Alternate clenching and spreading of the toes can be done in different positions—with the feet stretched forward on the floor, with the pressure on the outside of the foot; with the feet turned in and with them turned out. This exercise is an excellent guard against flat feet and is frequently given for dropped arches. It should be taken without any shoes on and can be practiced at any odd time—in bed or even in the bath!

# 13

# The Danger of Too-Early Pointe Work

Markova has been quoted as saying: "When I started to train in Pointe work—*you* had to do it, *not* the shoes." As a Cecchetti pupil, Markova wore the same soft, unblocked slippers throughout the entire class—for exercises at the barre, for work in the center of the studio and for pointe sequences. In this way, she learned that it was her foot, not her toe shoe, which enabled her to dance on pointe. It is the structure of the dancer's foot which governs her performance here—Markova has an unusually long big toe and it carries her entire weight when she is on pointe. Usually, it is the dancer with the square foot that enables her, on pointe, to stand on two, three or perhaps four toes, who is physically capable of executing all the virtuosi movements on pointe. The rather loose, over-arched foot will never be technically brilliant.

The square-footed dancer, with an arch that can be developed through careful training is more advantageously placed than the dancer who has toes that are too long in proportion to her instep. To become proficient and avoid injury the latter requires more help than can be supplied by the ordinary set of exercises; additional strength has to be given to her arches. Additional BATTEMENTS TENDUS may be sufficient or she may even require specific remedial exercises. One such exercise is to stand with toes and heels close together in the inward position, grip the ground with the toes, then propel the foot forward in a scuffling movement without raising it from the ground; do this with alternate feet, effecting a slow move forward.

There are two arches to a dancer's foot—the longitudinal tarsus, nearest the heel and the transverse metatarsus, near the toes; each must be developed evenly. Particularly the longitudinal arch must never be allowed to relax during barre and center practice, especially at the end of any movement of PLIÉ or FONDU. When the student is ready to go on to pointe the importance of this will be realized. It is just as necessary, but more difficult to build up the muscles controlling the transverse arch. If this is not done, with the passing of time, the feet will not maintain their correct and normal shape. Among other things, lack of strength in this region causes the enlarged toe joints from which so many dancers suffer.

The best long term method of achieving the desired strength in the muscles supporting the metatarsus is for the student to wear flat shoes for barre exercises, center practice and adage. Only when the muscles of the feet are reasonably developed should soft blocks be worn for this part of the class. Side practice is essential as a preparation for the more strenuous work in the center and it should be done in unblocked shoes. No foot can work well and be supple if it is restricted in heavy and unworkable pointe shoes with "wooden blocks" in the toes.

It has already been emphasized that the real pointe is the foot itself, not the shoe, which is only a covering. Constantly, the student must work to strengthen her instep (the longitudinal arch) to be able to work safely on pointe. The correct position is vital—when the foot is on pointe, the instep must be held straight over the toe, which must not be curled. The body must be held in a straight line with an absolutely straight back and the shoulders down. For the dancer, ankle strength is located on the inside of the foot and the student must have a strong ankle. Too many dancers fail to practice pointe on both sides; this particularly applies to PIROU-ETTES. This develops one foot more strongly than the other and is a bad thing.

Of the four basic POINTE movements, RELEVÉ and PIQUÉ are often performed incorrectly so that the dancer is in danger of injury when practicing turns on POINTE. So that the dancer gives herself a fair chance of performing correctly when she turns EN DEHORS, she must realize that RELEVÉ and PIQUÉ are exactly opposite movements. For the former, the toes are drawn toward the heel; for the latter the heel is thrust forward toward the toes. Fig. 7 shows the dancer, having correctly performed the RELEVÉ, turning on balance. Fig. 8, in which the dancer has substituted a PIQUÉ for the RELEVÉ, reveals a complete lack of balance. In Fig. 9, the dancer is on balance and shows correct line, having thrust the heel forward toward the toe. She has not done this in Fig. 10 and seems likely to fall.

Girls training as ballet dancers should avoid pointe work until they are assured that their feet are strong enough to attempt it. Permanent damage can be done to the feet if pointe work is attempted too soon. Some girls acquire the necessary strength sooner than others; it is not possible to make a definite statement as to what

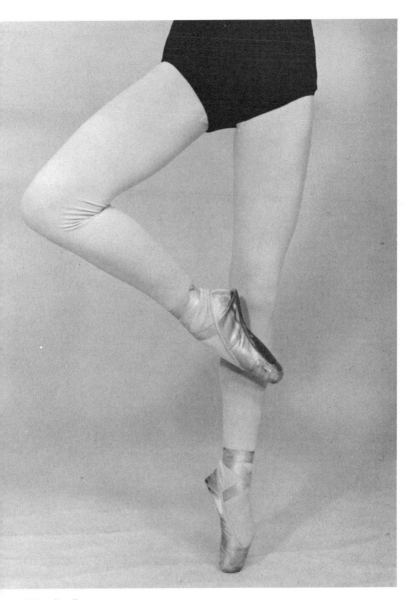

Fig. 7. Correct

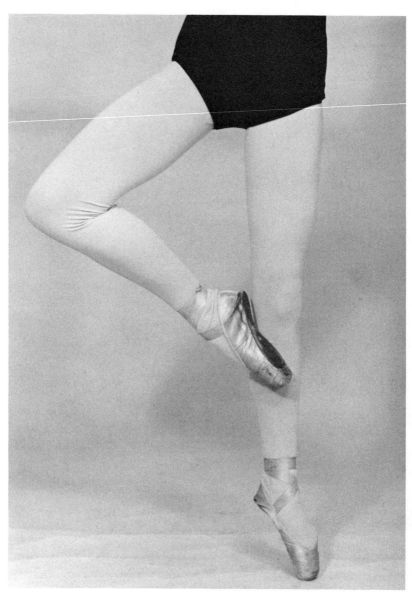

Fig. 8. Incorrect

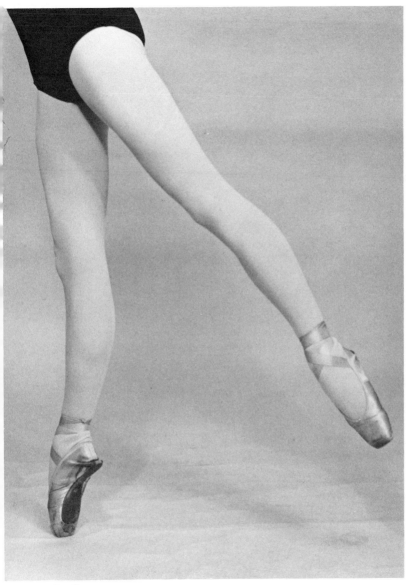

Fig. 9. Correct

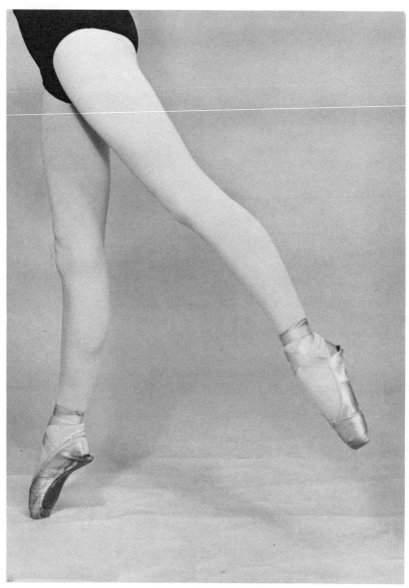

Fig. 10. Incorrect

stage in her training a dancer can attempt pointe work. It is an individual decision, made with the expert advice and assistance of an experienced teacher; it should not be attempted too early.

Pointe should be gradually practiced; only a little at first, such as a few ECHAPPÉES and RELEVÉS in the fifth position.* Plisetskaya was a dancer who represented the virtuosity of the Russian ballerina at its most fiery and glittering peaks; she tells the girl who is ready for pointe work, "You start with RELEVÉS in the five positions . . . . ." When a girl becomes a star like Plisetskaya, she commences her daily toe exercises with the RELEVÉ, the eternal and essential key to dancing on pointe. Before reaching this exalted stage, DEMI-POINTE work and more DEMI-POINTE work is the only way to have strong enough feet for the ultimate good of pointe work. Barre work will also strengthen the feet and legs besides improving balance— all dispensable to pointe work.

The correct position of the feet when actually on pointe is not the final achievement; the trained dancer knows and appreciates the importance of coming down correctly off pointe. Plates 8 and 9 show the dancer finishing a PAS DE BOURRÉE PIQUÉ; Fig. 11 is correct, No. 12 is incorrect. In the second case, there is a dropping in of the knee and the rolling of the ankle on the supporting foot can lead to development of the many muscles of the leg. Rolling over, especially when the weight of the body comes down, puts a strain on the cartilages of the knee joint and may lead to a tear or displacement of those structures.

At a more advanced stage, great care is required

---

* Rises in the first position are claimed to be a most important exercise as they indicate whether a child is strong enough for pointe work.

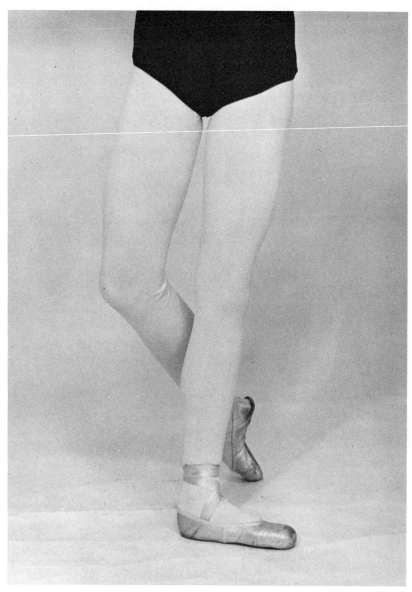

Fig. 11. Correct

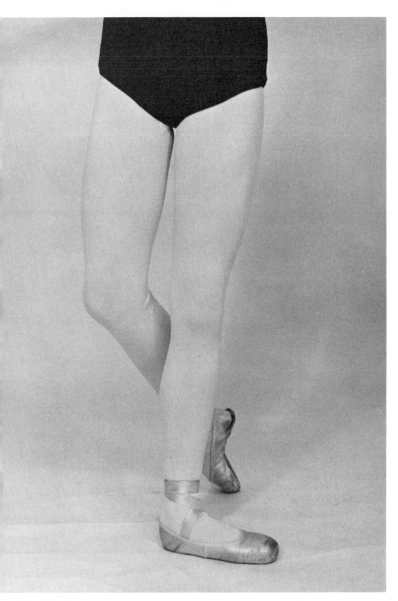

Fig. 12. Incorrect

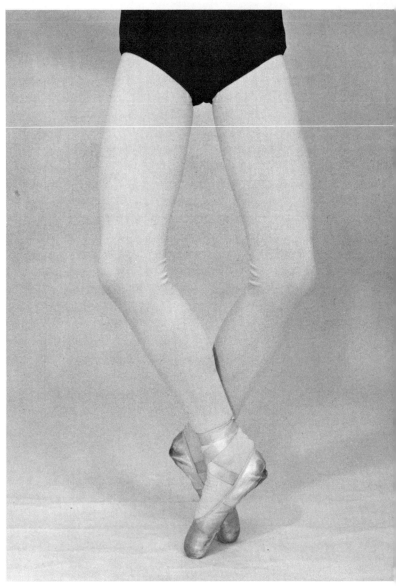

Fig. 13.

when jumping or hopping on pointe. The arch of the foot, together with the ankle, must be "clenched" and held tense; softness or relaxation here is dangerous. Fig. 13 shows a dancer just completing an ENTRECHAT QUATRE ON POINTE; one can plainly see the strain through the insteps. That physical effort must be confined to the insteps; any sign of strain in the rest of the body means that the dancer is not yet fit to perform this feat.

Pointe work should not be attempted until the body can support itself through possessing adequate strength in the muscles of the back and loins. More than that the student should understand right from the start that pointe work is really done with the muscles of the heels and not so much with the toes. To appreciate this, the use of the heel in BATTEMENT TENDU should not only be explained but insisted upon. In the same way, in BATTEMENTS FONDU, the function of the heel and the instep must be explained and practiced. The muscles and tendons of the heel must be strengthened and developed to cope with this work.

Sometimes, girls who are doing a lot of pointe work on hard floors suffer from a condition known as "dancer's heel." It manifests itself by pain above the calcaneous bone of the foot (at the Achilles Tendon area) and is caused by a bruising and swelling of those parts of the Calcaneous and Talus bones that pass over each other. To maintain balance, the knee has to flex a little when a dancer performs with this condition. Once bruised, this joint takes time to recover and rest is often the only remedy, as routine physiotherapy treatment sometimes has little effect.

Before leaving pointe work, it is fitting to consider

the vexing and frequently aired subject of very young children dancing on full pointe. There are still a few so-called teachers who allow children of five, six or seven years of age to "dance on the toes." It is a crime to put a child of five on pointe; the toe knuckles are underdeveloped and soft, their immature limbs, muscles and ligaments, cannot possibly support the extra strain entailed by pointe work. Permanent injury can result and the child's future as a real dancer can be considerably jeopardized. At best, the child when older will probably have to wear a double shank in her toe-shoe to give additional support to the metatarsal arch.

It can be claimed that Russia pays perhaps more serious attention to the training of a dancer than in any other country. It is instructive to note that pupils are not admitted to the Ballet Schools of Leningrad and Moscow until they are nine or ten years of age; they do not attempt pointe work for at least a year after their entry. Responsible bodies in Great Britain, such as the Royal Academy of Dancing or the Imperial Society's Classical Ballet Branch, do not give the slightest encouragement to early pointe work.* This indicates that no teacher can urge as an excuse for too-early pointe work, the desire to excel in examinations or competitions.

It has been suggested that mothers are very largely to blame; that they do not consider their children to have been properly taught until the infant can fumble through a "Rose Dance" on full pointe before an admiring, envious and equally ignorant group of friends. No teacher with a shred of self-respect for herself or

---

* They condemn it completely. These bodies do not expect pointe work in examinations till the child is thirteen in the case of R. A. D. and fourteen in the case of the Imperial.

her school would be a party to the risk involved to any child merely to avoid losing a pupil. The battle must be with those teachers who, for mercenary or unintelligent reasons, perpetuate this mistaken practice because of public ignorance or the doubtful wisdom of maternal pride. Mothers should not be entirely blamed; they are justified in assuming that they can entrust their children to a school or a teacher with confidence, if not technical knowledge.

The manufacturers of ballet shoes should not (and probably do not) manufacture blocked toe shoes smaller than those worn by the average child of about ten years of age.

Just in case any teacher or mother who has encouraged early pointe work feels that these dangers are being exaggerated, here are the views of three authorities, whose words should carry weight!

Dame Ninette de Valois, of the Royal Ballet School, has been quoted as saying:

"One of the two major defects that have ruined the chances of entry of many young dancers is too much early pointe work.

Children should not receive ballet training under eight years of age, and pointe work should be eschewed for the first two or three years; even then it should only be attempted by *children who have studied every day for two years.*"

An orthodedic surgeon, Mr. Sidney L. Higgs F.R.C.S., was a member of the Executive Committee of the Royal Academy of Dancing at the time of writing the following:

"I cannot condemn too strongly the practice of putting small children on the full pointe. As an orthopedic surgeon with some experience of the harmful effects which can result, I am of the opinion that young growing feet should not be subjected to this strain lest permanent damage and deformity should be caused, especially to the great-toe joints.

There is always, of course, some danger inseparable from ballet dancing and precautions must be taken to reduce this.

In the first place, only those children with sound, strong feet should be accepted. Secondly, pointe work should be deferred until growth is well advanced and, even then, it is essential that teachers should pay special and constant attention to correct performance and should check any tendency to "rolling" or to take weight over the inner borders of the feet and toes."

Margot Fonteyn knows from her own training under great masters, from her work with Karsavina and from her own experience that dancing on pointe for the young student is something which demands knowledge, care and attention. Miss Fonteyn says:

"Before going on Pointe the child should have at least two years of ballet training and she should not attempt Pointe work until about the age of nine. Young students should start Pointe work holding onto the barre, probably for the first year at least, and would strongly advise the use of a shoe with a flexible back."

Markova would not have a child use toe shoes until she is eight or nine or even older and not until she has had an extended period of pre-Pointe exercises and learned how to carry her weight with her entire body and not on the toes alone.

Shoes are vitally important; Pointe shoes only last a short time—the dancers of the Royal Ballet Company are said to be given at least eight pairs a month. One faulty batch can cause a lot of trouble. A toeshoe is a protection from the floor and not a support for the foot. The stronger the foot, the softer the shoe that can be worn. A foot in which the strength has been developed by exercises can tolerate lighter shoes. The strengthening of the feet in unblocked shoes, by careful and unremitting work on the Demi-Pointe is a vital necessity to every dancer.

No foot will ever fulfill what a dancer demands of it if that dancer "dances on her shoes and not her feet." The dancer should be conscious of the floor through her shoes; the tendency to use heavy blocks stuffed with plenty of cotton-wool is to be deplored although it may be very comfortable! If the toes become sore, they can be protected with lamb's wool inside the shoe; in hot weather spirit-gum in the tips of shoes will aid in retaining their shape and paper tissues will absorb perspiration.

Margot Fonteyn says: "I consider it very important to have a flexible sole, for it allows the maximum development of the foot itself, particularly of the sole of the foot. It is very important to exercise the whole foot and to be able to rise up to Pointe and down on the flat gradually passing through quarter, half and three-quarter Pointe on the way. A stiff sole impedes the proper exercising of the foot."

Fonteyn likes a soft block and a flexible sole but she expects support from her toeshoe and she wants it in that area of the foot running from the metatarsal arch to the toe. In her shoes, this support is provided by a small leather tongue placed under the inner sole.

With new shoes, it is sometimes best to select those

with medium hard box and a sole with double thickness to support the metatarsal arch. All new toe slippers, whether hard or comparatively soft, need to be broken in, in the same way as a walking shoe has to be worn several times before it becomes "a part of the foot." Many dancers simply walk around in a new pair of toe-shoes until the body's warmth softens the shoe and they begin to take on the shape of the feet. On the other hand, the heat of the body can make toeshoes too soft if they are overused; experienced dancers change their shoes for each ballet or their program. Remember, Pointe shoes require care and "doctoring" to make them last.

# 14

# Injuries to the Achilles Tendon

The Achilles Tendon can justly be termed "the main-spring of elevation," enabling the movement to finish with a smooth, controlled landing. Natural elevation is comparatively rare so that specific sets of muscles have to be developed to serve as a spring, lifting the body off the ground. Of course, there are also muscles of the knees and thighs that play an important part; together with the calf muscles which taper down into the Achilles Tendon, they must all receive adequate attention in the elementary stages of a dancer's training or there can be no perfect BALLON. The function of the Achilles Tendon is that of a strong elastic or a steel spring—it stretches and it contracts. The bigger the stretch the stronger becomes the contraction conditioning the push off the ground.

A strong elastic tendon is not only necessary for a perfect BALLON, it is also essential if the arduous strains placed upon this structure by dancing are not going to cause painful and limiting injuries. All forms of DEMI-PLIÉ (with pressure on the heels) should figure largely in daily practice; make sure that while the knees bend, the heels remain firmly on the ground. A quick, flexing of the knees does NOT serve the purpose! One of the best exercises is DEMI-PLIÉ in first position, giving it four counts, with a slight pause on each. Practice the exercise facing the BARRE; this will correct the tendency of the average pupil to push out the lower back.

BATTEMENTS FONDUS are also invaluable aids to elevation; they should be done both À TERRE and with RISE on DEMI-POINTE.

At the end of each class, go back to the BARRE and carry out the following mild limbering exercises. Face the wall in first position, slowly incline the body on the right side in DEMI-PLIÉ on the right foot, the other foot remaining straight. Then on the left side in the same way. The body should incline on the alternate sides as far as can be allowed by the stretch of the tendon and the support of the hands. The exercise must be done slowly and gently; younger pupils should only do it under the teacher's supervision.

Injuries to this region occur fairly frequently in physical activity and present a recurring source of trouble if not satisfactorily cleared up initially. This is because such activities involve movement of the feet, and such action must necessarily involve the Achilles Tendon as it is almost impossible to immobilize this structure and still satisfactorily move around enough for successful activity. The only gait which permits movement without pain to the Achilles Tendon is one of the extreme eversion of the foot, precluding balanced activity.

If one is to be guided by the majority of books dealing with trauma and sports injuries, it would appear that the most frequent injury to the Achilles Tendon is that of tenosynovitis. Tenosynovitis is the name of the condition in which inflammation attacks the sheath enclosing a muscle tendon. The smooth, inner lining of the sheath becomes roughened, causing tenderness and swelling as the delicate muscle fibers are "scraped" by the roughness.

The acceptance of this fact would seem to be difficult when it is considered that modern anatomical teaching categorically states that the Achilles Tendon has no sheath! That there is a painful and crippling condition involving the tendon cannot be denied, but it is not a true tenosynovitis and is labeled by different authorities as peritendinitis crepitans, tenovaginitis, or tendonitis. Many conditions affecting the Achilles Tendon are possibly inflammation of the bursa present between the tendon and the tibia, caused by the spread of the products of bruising from a damaged calf muscle, thus irritating the bursa and making it swell.

A bursa is a flattened pouch or bag containing fluid; these pouches are so placed as to provide a "cushioning" effect or to prevent damage, by friction, to a tendon when it continually passes over a bone.

Achilles Tendonitis, as the author knows the condition under discussion, frequently occurs in dancers because of the strain placed upon the tendon by the balance and stress of arduous dancing owing to the high degree of footwork involved over a lengthy active period. It would therefore seem to be due in the one case to stress and strain of sudden movement, while in the other because of prolonged strain over a period. The patient complains of sharp pain on movement and is forced to move in a flatfooted fashion; the pain is aggravated if there is a rotational strain with the foot fixed. There is exquisite tenderness along the length of the tendon, with one key spot that gives more pain than elsewhere. Sometimes a large spindle-shaped swelling can be found an inch from the attachment of the ligament.

The condition is usually caused by strain, but can also be non-traumatic, an irritative process affecting the tendon itself. The treatment has to be given by a physiotherapist and consist of deep-heating by short wave diathermy, deep friction-type massage, and rest from weight-bearing while carrying out a progressive routine of nonweight-bearing ankle exercises. At the conclusion of each session the ankle should be strapped with elastic adhesive plaster, using a sponge rubber heel and two strips of sponge rubber on either side of the tendon, the foot being in partial plantar flexion when being strapped. When using a high pressure technique, this treatment can be given thrice daily and will usually clear up the condition within three to five days. Should it not respond to this form of treatment, experience has shown that complete rest from the activity causing the condition must be ordered—it seems to make little or no difference during this period whether treatment is given or not! The condition clears up within about two to three weeks.

Home treatment, unless supplemented by sessions of short wave diathermy, does not seem to be very successful. It would appear that the condition does not react to any form of heat less penetrating than short wave diathermy, although bathing with alternate hot and cold water should be tried hopefully. The main consideration in both techniques is that the ankle should be adequately padded and strapped at all times when weight-bearing. If this is done, it will frequently be found possible to keep the dancer at full function while treating the condition.

A most effective exercise for pupils with tight Achilles Tendon lies in the use of an ordinary house brick or similarly sized wooden block. The pupil should stand in bare, or stocking feet, on the brick; front of toes level with forward edge of brick. Rhythmically, rise onto the toes and then allow the heels to drop until they touch the floor behind the brick.

# 15

# Injuries to the Knee Joint

When one considers the construction of the knee joint, it would initially seem to be one of the least secure joints in the body. The amount of leverage which can be brought to bear upon it is considerable, because it is formed from the two longest bones in the body, the femur and the tibia. The surfaces of these two bones which articulate together do not appear to be particularly suited to each other, and the joint possesses a very wide range of movement. All these factors tend to make the joint an insecure one, but, in reality, the joint is one of the strongest in the whole body, solely on account of the powerful ligaments which bind it together.

When confronted with any injury it is essential that the person responsible for treatment has some system of examination, in order that a diagnosis may be made and the necessary treatment instigated. There is no variety of injury to which this applies more strongly than that of damage to the knee joint. A large number of knee injuries demonstrate in their early stages symptoms identical with those of a torn cartilage, and it is therefore necessary to be able to differentiate between the lesser and the graver injury, thus allaying the patient's fears.

One such condition almost peculiar to dancers is the strain of an internal ligament of the knee joint—the medial coronary ligament. Caused by excessive rotation of the knee, the outward and visible signs of the condition is a puffy knee with obvious fluid. Tests elicit the "click" which usually denotes a torn cartilage and, indeed, the injury has all the earmarks of that condition. However, with heat and adequate, progressive quadriceps exercises, the knee will settle down in time and be as good as formerly.

First, a complete history of the condition must be made, exactly how it occurred, with the patient demonstrating the incident as far as possible. If the teacher was present when the injury occurred she will also have her own ideas on this point. Has the injury occurred previously? Has the knee ever "let the patient down"? Has it ever "locked" in semi-extension even for a split second? Has there ever been noticeable fluid around the joint? The significance of these questions is as follows: an old injury that frequently recurs indicates a possible cartilage lesion or an incompletely healed ligament tear. The sensation of "letting down" and locking tend to indicate a cartilage lesion, also. The presence of fluid on the knee joint indicates that there has been some actual violence involved, such as a blow, twist or wrench, because even quite a minor injury to this joint will cause the lining synovial membrane to become torn and to release a surplus of fluid, thus causing the joint to swell.

The joint should next be examined, signs of swelling sought, the discoloration of bruising should be looked for, and comparison made with the opposite knee joint. Marked differences may be found by this comparison. If swelling is insufficient to be conclusive, the joints of both legs should be gently felt to ascertain if there is a detectable "sponginess" of the injured joint. A diagnostic test to detect fluid on a knee joint is to press gently downwards with the palm of the hand on the supra-patella pouch, immediately above the kneecap; this action forces any fluid downwards into the lower part of the joint, and beneath the kneecap. The kneecap is now able to be gently "bounced" or "floated" by pressure with the tip of the finger. It is also possible to cause fluid to fluctuate from one side of the joint to the other, in the same way as one might press one side of a bladder filled with water and cause the water to surge over to the other side of the bladder, where it can be felt gently hitting against the hand.

Pain is of great importance when examining an injured knee, and it is sometimes possible accurately to diagnose the site of injury to this joint by means of a resisted extension of the knee joint. The patient is asked to straighten out his leg against the resistance of the operator's hand, the movement causing pain in the knee at the actual site of injury. Pain should be sought in two ways: one when it is caused by the patient's voluntary movement of the joint, and two, when it is elicited by means of pressure of the operator's fingers seeking the injury. A movement of the knee by the patient that causes pain will indicate that the actual injury is at the site of that pain. Pressure of the fingers will show at what level the external or internal ligaments of the joint are injured, or indeed any other of the superficial structures of the joint. Pain on pressure at the joint line indicates an injury to one or other of the cartilages, the joint line of the knee being a line drawn one centimeter below the lower limit of the kneecap, and continued around the knee at the level of the upper margins of the condyles of the tibia.

There are certain diagnostic tests which will prove almost conclusively that a particular injury that has been sustained. For example, in order to detect a strain or tear of either the external lateral or internal lateral ligaments, it is necessary to place one hand above the knee and the other at the ankle and "spring" the joint so that the suspected ligament is put on the stretch, thus causing pain to the injured man. A similar springing movement, but with one hand on the front of the leg above the knee and the other at the back of the ankle, will elicit pain in the rear of the joint and denote a strain of the rear fibers of the joint capsule. A straightening of the knee with the foot turned outwards that gives rise to pain on the inside of the joint, or an audible "click" denotes an internal cartilage lesion, while a similar movement with the foot turned inward that causes pain on the outside of the joint, or a similar "click" indicates an external cartilage lesion. This opinion is, of course, reinforced by a history of locking, fluid, etc. Rarely can it be said that all signs exist as in the textbooks.

No injury to the knee joint should ever be examined without taking a great deal of notice of the quadriceps muscles, the group that forms the muscle on the front of the thigh and which extends the knee joint. It is possible for a disabling injury to occur solely because this muscle group is lacking in strength or volume, which is a condition known as quadriceps insufficiency. This muscle group is the key to the knee joint, in that any lack of tone or size in them renders the knee joint inadequately supported, causing the knee to be insecure when stress is placed upon it. In turn, this encourages further wasting of the quadriceps, which causes the knee to be even more shaky, which is reflected in the quadriceps and so on, until it is hardly possible for the knee to remain steady for more than a few hours at a time. This vicious circle can only be broken into by the most conscientious and regular exercises of a progressive nature. The quadriceps can waste in seven days, lacking exercise, to a degree that will require six months' hard exercise to remedy. This being the case, it is obvious that in the event of any injury to the knee joint, it is essential that regular knee exercises are carried out in the form of static contractions (regular bracing of the knee thus hardening the muscles on the front of the thigh), straight leg lifting, and alternate flexing and extending of the knee joint while sitting with the legs dangling over the edge of a bed or table. Almost any injury to the knee will benefit by exercises of this sort. A specific DEVELOPPÉE exercise for strengthening the thigh muscles is to hold a DEVELOPPÉE, quickly lower and as quickly bring up the working leg without relaxing the thigh. The drop is very slight —only two or three inches—just a "wink" of the leg.

The monotony of quadriceps exercises can be broken by means of various forms of apparatus, which also has another use in that it enables progressive exercises to be carried out, weights of a known quantity being added at regular intervals. By the use of ropes and pulleys it is possible to devise an apparatus the one end of which is attached to the patient's foot by means of a strap; it then passes over two pulleys, and to a hook on the other end is attached bags of sand of varying weights. By means of alternate extension and flexion of the knee joint in a high-sitting position this weight is made to rise and fall, thus giving a known amount of resistance to the muscles working on the joint. Another method is to attach weights to the actual foot, while sitting in the same position and moving the limb in the same manner; the weighted boots used by weight lifters are ideal for this purpose.

One of the most common sports injuries to the knee joint is the strained ligament, either internal or external, the former occurring five times as frequently as the latter. The importance of this lies in the fact that the internal cartilage is attached to the internal ligament, which is not the case with the external cartilage and ligaments. Consequently, a severe strain of the internal ligament will frequently cause the cartilage to be torn at the same time. The tests for ligament strains have already been mentioned. There is a sudden, sharp pain on movement, particularly that of rotation of the knee, and a large degree of loss of function; there will frequently be later swelling and invariably a lot of fluid on the joint. The injured part must be supported at once with a firm pressure bandage, a pad of orthopedic felt placed directly over the site of injury and under pressure aids also. After a thirty-six hour period of nonweight-bearing during which time exercises must be carried out regularly, heat and massage is commenced and the exercises progressively increased.

An extremely severe injury is that of the rupture of a cruciate ligament, those two structures which, in each knee, connect the articular surfaces of the femur and the tibia. This injury occurs often at the same time as a torn cartilage, the complications associated with that condition frequently masking the more severe injury, that of the torn cruciate ligament. There are few surgeons who will undertake the complicated operation that involves grafting the actual cartilage onto the ruptured cruciate ligament, merely to enable a person to perform or dance, it being possible for a person suffering from this injury to carry out his daily life reasonably successfully. The weakened knee can be greatly strengthened by adequate quadriceps exercises, which indeed are absolutely essential if the patient is to carry on even his normal daily life.

The most publicized injury of the knee joint is that of the torn cartilage, a frequent but possibly overrated condition which it is now possible to cure completely in six to eight weeks, with adequate pre-and postoperative physiotherapy. Caused by a sudden twist of the knee with the foot firmly fixed by being planted on the floor, or by a twist of the lower leg with the thigh in an immovable position, the cartilage is torn loose from its attachments so that it becomes sometimes caught between the articular surfaces of the femur and tibia, thus causing the well-known locking of the joint. During dancing, similar aggravating movements might be RONDE DE JAMBE EN L'AIR and PETIT BATTEMENT. Once a cartilage has been torn and displaced it is inevitable that it will eventually have to be removed surgically. Even if it is replaced by a manipulation it will occur again with less strain, and so on until it is displaced almost at will. However, few doctors will remove a cartilage on the history of one displacement. Subsequently it is replaced by manipulative means, and a firm pressure bandage applied to control the inevitable effusion, or fluid outpouring. Quadriceps exercises follow until the knee is once again strong enough to bear the stresses and strains of active exercise.

As already mentioned, an outpouring of the synovial fluid invariably accompanies any injury to the knee joint, and it is therefore incorrect to label an injury "synovitis" and leave it at that. Synovitis is not a condition on its own but merely a reaction to injury, and its treatment is that of the underlying condition causing the effusion. It is not an easy task to disperse fluid once it has caused a knee joint to swell, and it frequently requires a well-planned combination of a number of methods. The application of hot towels is sometimes efficacious as is massage with the leg in an elevated position, thus aiding in the drainage of the fluid. A firm pressure bandage should be applied at all times when weight-bearing has to be done. As the majority of the fluid lies in the pouch above the kneecap, it is often a good measure to cut a piece of sponge, rubber or felt into a horseshoe shape, so that it fits around the kneecap, and then apply a normal pressure bandage over the top; the increased pressure aids drainage and dispersal. The application of a very firm and highly elastic rubber bandage to the knee joint and above, with the leg in elevation, and a series of contractions of the quadriceps carried out, will frequently disperse effusion. The constant rhythmic contraction and relaxation of the muscle group working on the joint causes the offending fluid to be "pumped" away.

Contusions or bruises suffered in the region of the knee joint are treated exactly as any other type of contusion, except that it is frequently necessary to apply a pressure bandage. The joint must be kept free by movement, and the quadriceps prevented from wasting by means of exercises. Excessive kneeling on hard floors can cause a soreness of the lower end of the kneecap which tends to prevent the sufferer from using her thigh muscles in their normal range. Pain is felt when the knee is fully straightened. A similar, but perhaps more serious condition, is caused by male dancers performing big turns that end on one knee.

There are a number of flattened pouches containing cushioning fluid in the region of the knee joint, known as bursae. One of these bursae frequently becomes inflamed, and as it is so placed that it is under the knee-cap, the condition that occurs is commonly known as housemaid's knee. The cause is irritation of the bursa, therefore the treatment is to remove the cause, which usually consists of kneeling on the offending knee so that in time inflammation occurs. In the chronic state removal of the bursa is the only cure and is quite a simple operation performed by a surgeon.

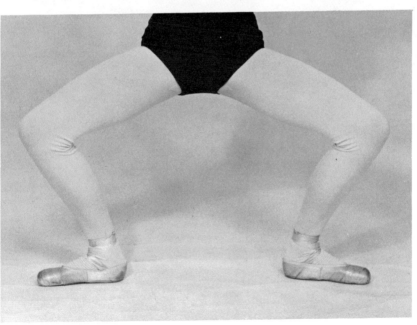

Fig. 14. Correct

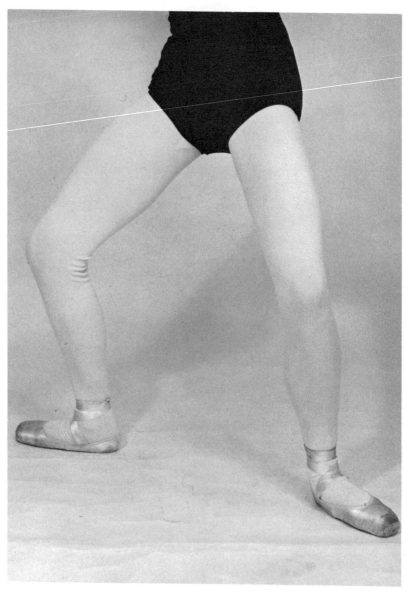

Fig. 15. Incorrect

At the commencement of the season, when dancers are unused to holding their hips externally rotated, they can cause soreness to the inner and lower border of the kneecap. More strain is taken by the inner side during knee-flexion exercises and in jumping, especially. Heat treatment helps to alleviate the immediate discomfort but, with the conviction that prevention is better than cure, other steps must be taken. Basically, it is a mechanical problem; the dancer must avoid turning the feet so far out until she can be sure of keeping her knees directly over her feet during PLIÉS. (See Figs. 14 and 15.)

The child must be made to understand from the first lessons how important it is to turn out from the hips with her weight over her little toes whatever the degree of turnout. Some children are capable of turning out fully from below the knee, keeping the thighs facing the front. This is often found in cases of poor teaching where the child has not been shown the importance of the turn out from the hip.

# 16

# The Trunk—Center of Strength

When a dancer is "placed" the muscles of the trunk have been so trained and developed that the physical demands of dancing can be handled with adequate muscular control and without loss of poise or presence. If muscular strength is lacking so that this control is absent then the dancer, away from the barre, will present a picture of unsteadiness, unbalance, uncoordination, plus neck and shoulder strain together with a complete lack of poise and presence. Such a situation presents a field wide open to injury.

The true strength of a dancer lies in the muscles of her trunk; the constantly building-up of these muscle groups must always be a prior consideration. The teacher and the student must be familiar with them and their role, together with an understanding of the way in which the limbs are attached to the trunk. Thus, the shoulder is attached to the back of the trunk and should never be allowed to drop forward; the legs are placed in front of the body and the turn-out has to get them placed as far as is humanly possible toward the back. This means that years of patient practice ensure the knees being bent at the finish of a step with the bend restricted to the knee and not passing along the thigh so that the trunk is bent forward and the buttocks protruding.

The rib cage forms the upper two-thirds of the trunk, going all the way round to the spine. During classical exercises the rib cage should be held level and slightly contracted. When told to "lift your ribs" the student does so in the front but drops them at the back; this causes a lack of control of the spinal muscles together with a relaxation of the diaphragm. The chest must always be lifted and expanded.

There is a common saying in athletics that "a runner is as good as his guts." Ignoring the implied courage factors the saying emphasizes the importance of a powerful set of abdominal muscles to anyone participating in active physical exercise. The dancer should ensure that not only the vertically-running Rectus Abdominus muscles and the corset-like Transversalis muscle are built up but also the External and Internal Oblique Abdominal muscles at the sides of the trunk. This can be done by including trunk twisting and side-flexion together with straight trunk or leg raising movements. Floor limbering will strengthen the lower abdominal muscles as well as giving flexibility to the spine. Strain is taken from the legs and the poise of the body is given a "lightness" that is missing when the student lets her trunk "sit" into the hips with slack lower abdominal muscles.

The muscles of the back are brought into play when the student endeavors to obtain maximum length in the space between the hipbone and the lowest rib without allowing a shoulder lift to creep in. This particular muscular contraction can be made during elevation exercises when the student alights after a jump; the weight of the trunk never being allowed to pass below the hip.

*All* the various parts of the body are equal in importance to the dancer—but some are more equal than others! Having said that the abdominal muscles are all-important we will now say that the spine is a vital part of a dancer's body. Katherine F. Wells, Ph.D., in her book "KINESIOLOGY" has written:

"If one were faced with the problem of devising a single mechanism that would simultaneously:

(1) Give stability to a collapsible cylinder.

(2) Permit movement in all directions, yet always return to the fundamental starting position.

(3) Support three structures of considerable weight —a globe (the head), a yoke (the shoulder girdle), and a cage (the chest and abdomen).

(4) Provide attachment for numerous flexible bands and elastic cords.

(5) Transmit a constantly increasing weight to a rigid basin-like foundation.

(6) Act as a shock absorber for cushioning jolts and jars.

(7) Encase and protect a cord of extreme delicacy, he would be faced with a task of staggering immensity. Yet the spinal column fulfils all these requirements with amazing efficiency. It is at the same time an organ of stability and mobility, of support and protection, of resistance and adaptation. It is an instrument of great precision, yet it is of robust structure. Its architecture and the manner in which it performs its many functions are worthy of careful study. From the kinesiologic point of view, we are interested in the spine chiefly as a mechanism for maintaining erect posture and for permitting movements of the head, neck and trunk."

It can be a tower of strength or a broken reed; from the

spine comes balance and strength, leading to good carriage and poise; ELEVATION and all PIROUETTES require strong backs. Only a flexible back can be a strong back; flexibility of the spinal column can be gained through exercises that loosen and control the vertebral muscles. Mainly, they are exercises for stretching and relaxation; rigidity in the back and shoulders is harmful to the moving body. Suppleness gives a balanced breadth and extension, recovery from which is gradual and not forced or jerked.

A badly poised head is a great handicap to a dancer as it usually indicates lack of strength or control in a movement. A head incorrectly poised usually accompanies the poor stance and carriage emanating from a weak back. The traditional barre as used in all ballet classes is excellent training for the achievement of strength and control in the back. In addition, the dancer needs a certain amount of limbering, particularly floor limbering, to gain the vitality, rebound and flexibility that add up to strength. From this strength comes the well-poised and proudly carried body that brings style and dignity to a dancer.

This poise is the principal reward gained by the child who does not hope to become a professional dancer. One class per week for ten years will enable a child to control her body and produce a degree of poise unable to be gained from any other form of physical activity.

Every word so far written in this chapter is probably familiar to the experienced teacher, who uses these factors to bring about a polished and competent performance in her students. There is another light in which they must be viewed—prophylactic. Muscular strength and posture compatible with the physical activities undertaken are the strongest weapons in the army of injury-prevention. The very nature of their intense activity renders dancers particularly injury prone and the trunk is an area possessing innumerable weaknesses. Dancers work in a very wide and full range of movement; the twisting, turning, bending and stretching give a mobile spine which, conversely, probably encourages that modern malady—the "slipped disc." On the other hand, the enhanced muscular strength and increased joint movement probably prevents disc lesions—almost for the same reasons that can cause them!

A girl will find that she has low back pain because of the overextension of her spine in ARABESQUE. The simple answer is not to force all the movement at the bottom of the spine (Fig. 16), but to spread the extension through all the spinal joints. Male dancers have continually to lift and carry their partners, either on their shoulders or in their outstretched arms. Strains of spinal muscles, "slipped discs" and early degenerative arthritis can result unless they have been instructed in correct ways of lifting, avoiding excessive bending back of the lower spinal area (Fig. 17 and 18). The men should also be given strengthening exercises for the arms and shoulder-girdles, thus taking some of the strain off the spine and trunk generally.

The hip joints sometimes give trouble to the dancer. In a movement where the dancer has to lift the leg sideways and turn it INWARDS instead of the usual outward rotation, pain is experienced and a tender area is felt just above the outer "knob" of the joint (the Greater Trochanter). This is caused by inflammation of a bursa (a shock-absorbing, friction-preventing bag of fluid) placed under the attachment of one of the buttock

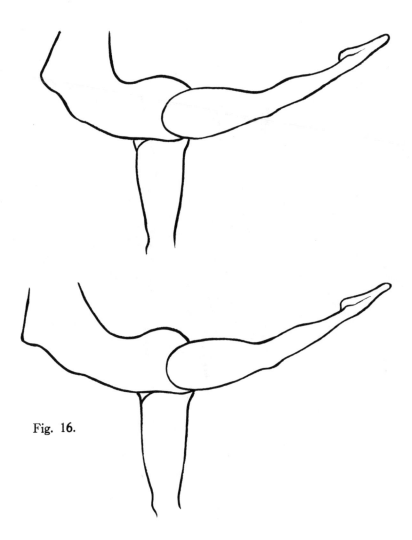

Fig. 16.

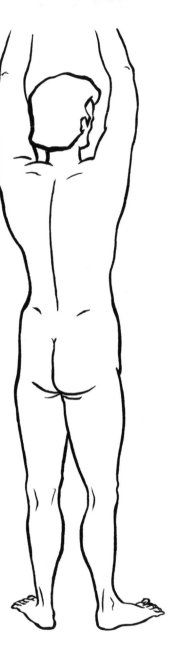

Fig. 17. Correct

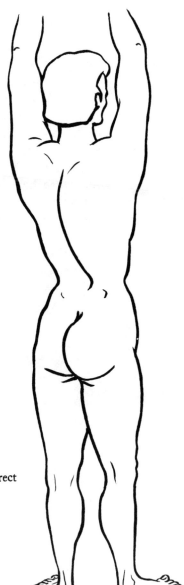

Fig. 18. Incorrect

muscles. A similar bursa in front of the hip joint can cause pain on flexion of the hip and when the leg is turned inwards. An injection of hydrocortisone is nearly always successful in clearing up this condition; otherwise rest will help.

The muscles on the inside of the thigh (the Adductors) are sometimes strained in the very wide range of hip movements performed by dancers. The painful point is often right up in the groin. Deep heat, such as short wave diathermy is required and the muscle must be progressively stretched by placing the inside of the foot of the injured leg on the seat of a chair and bending the knee of the other leg outwards, thus stretching the muscle group.

# 17

# The Trunk—Backache
# and the Slipped Disc

One of the greatest medical mysteries of today is the amazing increase in the incidence of backache. Popularly labeled "slipped disc" it is a sudden and temporarily crippling condition that seems to be brought on by many of the most frequent and apparently innocuous movements of everyday life. It is a definite clinical entity that can be held responsible for more than 90 percent of all painful symptoms in the lower back. Now knowing the symptoms to be caused by an underlying disc lesion, it automatically follows that twenty or thirty fancy names are now correctly grouped under the one title, thus giving the impression that there are twenty or thirty times as many slipped discs! Even so, this title is something of a misnomer in that sometimes an initial dislocation (subluxation) of the disc occurs and very quickly goes back into a harmless position. This "self-reduction" can be effected by a movement of the patient's or even a cough. The back muscles, in an effort to prevent more damage go into a spasm of cramp to fix the spine, the resultant pain and fixation due to this intense spasm. The most effective treatment consists of manipulations that break down the "matting" together of muscle fibers (adhesions) that have resulted from the spasm. It is a condition that may creep up insidiously upon the sufferer or it can strike suddenly with all the dramatic shock of a bedside telephone ringing in the dead of night!

This apparently troublesome structure, the intervertebral disc—where does it repose, of what is it made, and is its presence essential? It consists merely of a ring of fibro-cartilage surrounding a pulpy center. Cartilage, or gristle, is a tough bluish-white substance of firm consistence but elastic, yielding readily to pressure or torsion, but recovering its shape when the constraining force is removed. It possesses a firm ground-substance or matrix into which is introduced bundles of white fibrous connective tissue, giving the required additional strength. This cartilage is a tissue serving chiefly to support and connect other structures of the body; thus it has to be tough, resistant, less brittle and more flexible than other tissues.

The vertebrae forming the spine move about on each other, their frontal bony mass or body being separated from each other by the thick circular pads of fibro-cartilage (intervertebral discs). The discs act as a sort of cushion or shock absorber to break the "jar" arising from a sudden concussion of the vertebral column, and also bind the vertebrae into a column which is resistant but at the same time flexible.

Slipped discs are very easy to understand because the disc obeys the simplest mechanical laws. It will move in any direction in which it is pushed, as it consists of inert material and lies unattached within every spinal joint. It is subject to two forces: the first, centrifugal, due to the compression of body weight and muscular contraction, and the second, to whatever inclination or slant the adjacent joint surfaces adopt at any moment.

Disc lesions can only occur within the actual vertebral joint and, even then, it is only when the displaced part protrudes directly backwards or backwards and to one side simultaneously. The resulting symptoms are only caused by pressure on adjacent sensitive structures. Such structures only lie to the rear and rear/side of the joint —in the rear is the dura mater, the membrane lining the inner spinal cavity, and to rear and side are the nerve roots emerging from the spine. It is only impingement on these structures that gives rise to the patient's symptoms.

The disc's outer ring of cartilage may crack under certain circumstances; this causes no symptoms until such a fragment becomes dislodged, giving rise to a sudden, dramatic onset of pain. A similar situation occurs when the cartilage (or meniscus) of the knee joint is displaced. The pulpy center, or nucleus, can sometimes extrude, occurring slowly and gradually, and gives rise to the backache that begins insignificantly and insidiously; such an extrusion can occur without any prior damage to the outer ring.

When the protruding disc is pressing on the dura mater (lining membrane of the spinal column) it can cause pain to be referred to other parts of the body—a disc lesion at the 5th lumbar level can cause pain down to the buttocks or any part of the thigh. This "referred" pain is accompanied by local deep tenderness, but this tenderness is a result not a cause, and therein lies the idea of "fibrositis," "myalgic spots," "trigger areas," "nodules," all of which are frequently blamed for the local pain.

This is a completely incorrect diagnosis based on inadequate examination of joint and muscle function and the insistence of the patient as to the site of his pain.

Such an error is a blessing to the manufacturers of rubbing oils and smelly embrocations which do little more than give a transient warmth to the part being rubbed. The effects of massage with embrocation are merely the effect of massage.

It is also possible to sustain a slipped disc in parts other than the lumbar spine (lower back). The patient can awake with a stiff neck and pain in the area of one shoulder blade. Marked limitation of movement is noticed predominantly in one direction. This decreases as the attack subsides, the displaced disc spontaneously edging back into its rightful plance. Recurrence is common, particularly if sleeping on a pillow of incorrect thickness. (One that prevents the head lying level during rest). Intermittent pain in the shoulder blade is sometimes experienced, and is followed by several weeks' severe pain in the upper arm, often with numbness and tingling sensations in the fingers. The pain is worse at night and prevents sleep. The condition is sometimes incorrectly called brachial neuritis, whereas it is really the upper limb parallel to the sciatica of the leg.

A pain in the middle of the back is exactly like lumbago, but higher up. It is caused by bending or twisting when lifting a weight, and recovery is much quicker than in the lower back, two or three days in bed doing the trick. It is rare to have a severe attack of thoracic disc lesion; a few days' pain is followed by a few weeks' freedom, the attacks being related to prolonged flexion of the spine or compression of the affected joint.

A cough will cause back pain in lumbago and sciatica a deep breath hurts when the condition is in the middle of the back, but a deep breath or cough seldom hurts when the pain is in the neck.

Research has indicated that there is one particular type of strain that produces prolapse of an intervertebral disc, and, conversely, that it is nonsense to suggest that all heavy work places the worker in jeopardy. Medical notes invariably record that the patient strained his back while lifting, but these notes rarely mention that at the initiation of the moment of lift the spine was in the position not only of flexion, but also of slight rotation and flexion to one side, thus, in rising the spine was therefore brought back to the straight position by a corkscrew motion. While lifting, the man is making a voluntary effort to straighten his back against the resistance of the weight of the article being lifted, this resistance being applied indirectly through the arms. So it can be said that in a disc injury the force is deliberately produced by a voluntary muscular effort. You can sprain joints in your back just as you can sprain an ankle, and the easiest way is to lift something when you are leaning forwards.

If a healthy individual is asked to bend and touch his toes and then recover to the erect position, he will be found to maintain regular breathing, probably exhaling during bending and inhaling on straightening the back. When a man is asked to raise a heavy weight, he bends freely but rises against the resistance of the lifted weight. In these circumstances the man usually exhales bending; then there is a preliminary intake of breath, the breath is held at the initiation of the lift and is released after inertia has been overcome and the movement of straightening the spine has begun.

This momentary holding of the breath means that the various parts of the respiratory system are fixed; the diaphragm, being the lowest part and being attached to the first three lumbar vertebrae, causes them to be held immobile. This means that movement of the lower back, as in straightening up, occurs first in the low lumbar region which causes maximum pressure on the lowest two discs in the lumbar area, thus forcing the discs to bulge slightly backwards.

When the man begins to straighten his back against the resistance of the weight, he often slightly rotates his spine and deviates a little to one side. This causes movement of the lower two lumbar vertebrae so that they nip the bulging disc in a grinding movement with maximum pressure exerted to one side of the mid-line according to whether the man is inclined to the right or left.

The spinal joints most subject to disc lesions are the fourth, sixth and seventh cervical and the fourth and fifth lumbar—the very areas of the spine constructed in such a fashion as to have the most pronounced curves. These curves mean that the joint space is wider in front than behind, which ensures that a slight pressure, directed forward, is constantly exerted on the intervertebral disc during weight-bearing and means that the body has to be well flexed before the back of the joint is wider than the front. If the joint surfaces lie parallel, as they tend to do in the flat-backed patient, a slight degree of trunk-flexion begins at once to squeeze the disc backwards, and at full trunk-flexion the amount of narrowing of the part and gaping of the back of the joint is greater than in his fellows.

A large number of the sufferers from low back pain do not actually have a disc lesion when they are examined, although they undoubtedly did have one in the initial stages of their trouble. This disc protruded and then, for one reason or another, spontaneously went back into its position—at the onset of pain caused by the disc displacement the muscles of the lower back went into a spasm, and they became rigid in an attempt to "scaffold" the back against an incautious, painful movement. Then ensued a vicious circle, in that the muscular spasm forced the patient to move in a stiff, timid fashion that in time became painful, the pain in turn causing the patient to move in a stiff, timid fashion! This circle can only be broken into by manipulation (either self-induced by exercise or carried out by a physiotherapist or doctor) to break down the adhesion of muscle fibers caused by the spasm, and then exercises to maintain the mobility of the back and return it to its original pristine condition.

A disc lesion should be treated as a medical emergency, approached by the doctor with a sense of urgency, and afforded a high priority. Unfortunately, this is rarely the case, and a protracted sequence of events begins that frequently ends, after months of pain, loss of working time and consequently loss of money, with the patient turned into an apprehensive semi-neurotic, self-condemned to nothing more than the lightest exertion for the rest of his life. If a person with a fracture or a dislocation is immediately rushed into the casualty department of the nearest hospital—then a disc sufferer should be afforded the same treatment because he, too, has a dislocation within one of the most vulnerable joints of his body.

When a disc "slips" all possible future trouble is only obviated if it is returned to its position as soon as possible. This means that the patient will lose his symptoms almost at once, and, more important, needless stretching of protective structures around the disc will be reduced to a minimum. These structures (ligaments) are the only bar to the disc further protruding and causing pressure on the nerve root, after the initial irritation of the lining of the spinal column (dura mater), giving rise to sciatica of long duration. The period of disability for a disc-sufferer can almost be said to be in direct ratio to the speed with which the condition is treated.

The manipulations that reduce discs consist of a carefully controlled series of movements on the patient, who cooperates with the manipulator throughout by informing him verbally, and with movements, of his reaction to each step. It is not a hasty, routine set of forced manipulations performed on an anaesthetized patient, who is therefore unable to give any immediate indication as to the effects of the various movements. It is almost painless and can be dramatic in its effects, the patient crawling into the clinic and literally running out! A man can return to work the same day following manipulation, and successful results can be obtained in two or three treatments.

Sciatica, a pain that runs down the leg sometimes to the very toes, is caused by a "soft disc" when the pulpy nucleus or center of the disc oozes out over (or through) the disc's hard, fibrous rim. Sciatica is a progression of backache and is caused by the protruding portion of disc moving sideways to press upon the spinal nerve root rather than the lining membrane of the spine, the dura mater. Its onset is slow and insidious. It is treated by means of "traction"—a stretching of the spine.

The patient lies on a couch to which is affixed a screwed apparatus that extends in a manner similar to a vise being opened. Attached to the apparatus is a padded set of straps, which fasten around the patient's hips; another set fasten around his chest and are bound to the far end of the couch. When the screw is extended, the lower straps pull on the patient's hips against the fixed straps around the chest—thus the area between the straps is stretched. Admittedly, it sounds horrible, and patients jocularly compare it to the rack of Spanish Inquisition days—but it does not hurt in any way, apart from a possible slight discomfort due to the tightness of the straps. If a patient is put into traction with sciatic pain running down his leg, he will find that the pain noticeably recedes as traction is applied. During traction, the patient apparently stretches about six inches —this is purely transitional!

Traction is not so speedy in its results, but is the only treatment that will have any effect on sciatica or a soft disc lesion. It follows that if a hard fragment of displaced disc can be "clicked" back into place, then a soft, pulpy protrusion, having the consistency of wet sand, can only "ooze" back into place. To allow this to happen, the two vertebrae from which the disc has emerged have to separate, the increasing of the distance between them not only enlarging the space into which the pulp can now return but also creating suction.

Traction has two effects—first, it separates the vertebrae and allows the disc to be squeezed back into place; second, it tautens the ligament running lengthways down the back of the spine, causing pressure on the disc protrusion and slowly pushing it back. Traction should be carried out daily, in thirty-minute sessions, until the pain is relieved and symptoms vanish.

At the outset, some disc lesions are so acute, causing such a high degree of pain, that no form of physical treatment is possible, so that the sufferer has no alternative but to lie prone and immobile in bed. This is the traditional treatment and the best one in the early stages until, aided by pain-killing drugs, the condition settles down enough to permit physical treatment to be tolerated. The patient remains in bed for a few days, avoiding movement that elicits pain, particularly bracing his back when coughing. This rest should not be confused with the conservative and optimistic putting to bed for weeks that some doctors inflict upon their patients. It is no substitute for physical treatment and is only used to quiet down the condition sufficient for more active measures to take place. Rest in bed is an admission of defeat and can take weeks or months to be effective, if at all. The bed should be hardened to prevent sagging of the back, also prevented by a small pillow in the small of the back, and toilet facilities must be provided so that the patient does not have to get out of bed or sit up.

There are certain indications in disc lesion that justify what is known as an epidural injection of anaesthetic in the lower back. The introduction of the anaesthetic into the offending area will relieve the effects caused by the pressure of the displaced disc on surrounding structures, particularly after the disc has been reduced. This is dramatically effective, and the patient is able to walk home thirty minutes after the injection.

When routine measures fail, or sometimes even in conjunction with them, a course of back exercises is prescribed. As mentioned before, when the trouble is due to adhesions following a disc lesion, these exercises are of great benefit, but when a disc is actually out of position the advantages of exercises are rather debatable. Sufficient to say that in the latter case they should be confined only to back extension exercises (arching of the lower back), and in neither case should forward flexion of the trunk be included in the scheme.

Some of the most successful but awe-inspiring forms of treatment are given to the neck to reduce a cervical disc lesion. This can be dramatically replaced to give 90 percent improvement at once by means of manual manipulation. It is essential that strong traction to given to the neck at the same time. This is done by the operator, with one hand under the patient's chin, as he lies supine, and the other under the back of the head, laying his weight backwards and pulling. In this way, the joint surfaces are separated to allow the disc to return, aided by the push of a tautened ligament; the patient's pain vanishes and he can permit manipulatory movements that hitherto would have been impossible owing to muscular spasm.

Prolonged traction, if required, can also be given to the neck, something in suspension with the patient sitting up, head encased in a harness suspended from an overhead apparatus—frightening perhaps, but painless and very effective. A collar of felt and cardboard is occasionally worn to give a measure of traction, maintain a good position of the neck to encourage reduction, and also prevent injudicious movements. Spontaneous cure of cervical disc lesions can occur after two to four months, during which period the patient should take analgesics to aid him at night when the pain is worse.

Simple aids consist of wearing high heel shoes when suffering from sciatica—"flatties" stretch the sciatic nerve and aggravate the condition. Dancers in a touring company sleep in a variety of beds, some soft, some sagging and some hard. This is not exactly condusive to helping the back that has a tendency to ache! A bed that sags is the worst and should be supported by a piece of wood, a tray or even a folded coat. The back-ache sufferer can often obtain relief by laying on the floor with a small cushion or folded towel supporting the low-back curve.

When one considers the suppleness of a child's spine and the twists and contortions that it makes during a normal day's youthful activities, it is not surprising to learn that disc lesions can occur in children. A reason-ably accurate description of the relevant symptoms has been recorded by a girl of eight, and the full range of signs of pain in the leg, limitation of back movement and deviation of the spine (postural deformity) have been noted in both sexes between the ages of twelve and fifteen.

Such occurrences should not be unexpected because there is good reason to think that disc lesions are born with the individual and therefore date from childhood. Being congenital, a family history of backache can often be traced, attacking all the children in one generation and members of three or four generations. When an adolescent indicates her choice of a dancing career, she should be asked to think again if both her parents suffer from lumbago or sciatica.

Patients can often recall certain positions or activi-ties in childhood that invariably brought on low-back pain, and will ruefully admit that they were always considered to have a back that was "weak." In this respect, girls seem to outnumber the boys!

Sciatica is very rare before the age of eighteen but a minor strain to the back, or a period of bed rest with some other illness, will set up a low-back pain in the adolescent lasting some days or weeks. The youngster gradually realizes that it has disappeared, but it frequently recurs and again abates quickly. Such a sequence of events often gives rise to grave, incorrect treatment that can have far reaching effects in the patient's later life. Labeled "postural pain," a routine of exercise is ordered, guided by aesthetic considerations, whereas the alleviation of the present pain and the prevention of future backache should be the prior aim.

# 18

# Injuries to the Upper Extremity

The shoulder girdle is composed of three separate joints: that beween the upper and outer part of the sternum or breastbone and the inner end of the clavicle or collarbone, that formed by the outer end of the clavicle and the inner margin of the acromion process of the scapula and finally, the joint formed by the hemispherical head of the humerus and the shallow glenoid cavity of the scapula. These joints are known respectively, as the sternoclavicular, and the acromioclavicular and the shoulder joint.

The strength of these joints mainly depends upon their ligaments which limit the amount of movement in each joint, the joints being maintained mostly by the tendons of the muscles working on the joints. In the case of the actual shoulder joint, the relative sizes of the two articular surfaces and the looseness of the articular capsule enables the joint to enjoy remarkably free movement in all directions. Extremely important in the treatment of any injury to the shoulder girdle is the biceps muscle, formed by two distinct "heads" which are attached to the scapula above and to the back of the head of the radius below. Therefore, by its connection with both the shoulder and elbow the muscle harmonizes the action of the two joints and acts as an elastic ligament in all positions. This means that the joint is provided with a ligament which is not only of great power in resisting movements that would harm the joint, but which will also yield spontaneously when necessary.

Shoulder injuries are fairly common in physical activity. Fractures, ligament strains and contusions occur while the shoulder joint is more frequently dislocated than any other joint owing to its construction and the freedom of movement which it enjoys, as well as in consequence of its exposed situation. It is very essential that the teacher has a definite system of examination when confronted with an injury to the shoulder girdle so that she can rule out the more serious types of injury. A suggested method is as follows:

(a) Observation. While the clothing or equipment worn will preclude direct vision, it is possible to detect the way in which the injured shoulder is "carried," how the arm is used and the sufferer's attempts at protecting the injured part. There will always be a favoring of the uninjured arm, the man will try to perform tasks with his left arm, for example, that he would normally carry out with his right arm, and he will show a definite inability to use the injured limb correctly and freely. Also look for visible deformities.

(b) Feel. By means of gentle probing with the fingertips it is possible to detect tenderness, deformity, abnormal mobility, particularly along the clavicle. If these symptoms or signs are not present in the region of the collar bone it is possible to rule out three common injuries to that region: (i) dislocation of the sterno-clavicular joint, (ii) dislocation of the acromi-clavicular joint and (iii) a fractured clavicle. The presence of the three symptoms of deformity, tenderness and abnormal mobility in the region of the shoulder joint will indicate a dislocation of the head of the humerus. Having ruled out the more serious injuries, the less serious types such as sprains and contusions can be discovered and readily treated.

(c) Muscle and Joint Functional Tests. The shoulder girdle will move through the following ranges: flexion, extension, abduction, adduction, inward rotation, outward rotation and a combination of all these movements —circumduction. The teacher should endeavour to gently move the joint through its full range, without any assistance from the patient. The patient should then be told to move the joint through its fullest range without any aid. Finally, the teacher should again grasp the limb and instruct the patient to move it through its various ranges, at the same time applying a very slight degree of resistance to each movement. From pain incurred by these movements it will be possible to ascertain at what particular point the injury lies and the specific muscles or ligaments involved.

A fall on an outstretched hand can cause the clavicle to become fractured, the force of the blow usually being transmitted along the long axis of the bone which causes the clavicle to be fractured rather than displaced. The signs are pain, shock, inability to move the arm on the side of injury, the head will frequently be tilted to the affected side, and the patient will hold his hand under his elbow to support the arm. The area of the injury will be tender, there will be swelling and tenderness along the line of the bone, while it is sometimes possible to feel displaced bony fragments. All of these signs will rarely be present at one and the same time, but enough of them will be detectable to enable the teacher to know whether or not she is confronted with a fractured clavicle.

The immediate treatment is to send for a doctor, after applying some form of support, which may either take the form of a figure-eight bandage around both shoulders pulling them back into a braced position, or else the St. John's-type bandage formed by two slings, one under the elbow and up over the shoulder to support the arm, while the other one is around the arm and the body, with a pad under the armpit. Support is worn for about three weeks and is not removed until there is free arm and shoulder movement without pain. During the first week it is important to exercise all joints of the limb from shoulder to fingers thus preventing stiffness, and the arm must be supported throughout by a triangular sling. At the end of the first week the joints of the shoulder girdle are gently exercised to maintain mobility. After three weeks, heavier exercises involving some form of light resistance may be given to redevelop the muscles of the shoulder girdle. It is stated that these particular muscles waste more rapidly than any others in the body, with the exception of those working the knee joint. And, as has already been stated, the biceps muscle tendon acts as a ligament to the shoulder joint and the tendons of other muscles around the joint are responsible for maintaining the joint, so the importance of these exercises can be rapidly seen.

It has already been stated that the shoulder joint is more readily dislocated than any other joint, the most frequently encountered form of dislocation being that which occurs when the head of the humerus assumes a position in front of the neck of the scapula, beneath its coracoid process, and is therefore named the subcoracoid dislocation. The signs are those of pain, tenderness, shock, the shoulder is "flattened" and its normal contour is lost, the elbow is unable to touch the same side of the body and the patient cannot touch the opposite shoulder. It is also possible to feel the head of the humerus in its abnormal position. After the dislocation has been reduced by a doctor a large pad is placed in the armpit and the limb is supported in a sling or a collar and cuff of bandage for two to three weeks. During this period exercises are given to maintain the mobility of the shoulder joint and the muscles of the arm, but no shoulder movements should be given for the first six days, and then only of a supported type.

There are certain complications which must be watched when dealing with a dislocation of the shoulder. The first of these is a paralysis of the deltoid muscle, caused by the nerve supplying that muscle (the circumflex nerve) to be nipped as it winds around the neck of the humerus, the danger signal being that the joint becomes stiff or the deltoid muscle wastes. Other complications include a fracture to the head of the humerus, an injury to the brachial plexus of nerves which will involve the majority of the muscles of the upper extremity, and recurrent dislocation. The latter condition indicates that the joint is readily dislocated with little force being applied, the best known remedy being surgical reconstruction of the joint.

Sprain of the ligaments of the joints of the shoulder girdle are caused by a direct blow on the shoulder, a fall on to the elbow or outstretched hand, or a sudden backward wrench of the shoulder. There is swelling and localized tenderness over the joint, and a marked loss of function and power of the arm. A support such as a sling, or an adhesive plaster strapping over a sponge rubber pad placed on the shoulder, must be applied for the first forty-eight hours after injury. Then follows the usual treatment for a sprain: heat with massage and exercise. Under no circumstances should the dancer be permitted to resume her activities until she has been put through the most rigorous tests to prove that her shoulder movements are normal and without pain.

In the rehabilitation of injuries to the shoulder girdle it is essential to maintain abduction (the lifting of the arm sideways from the body) and outward rotation of the shoulder joint. Injuries to the shoulder region are usually extremely painful particularly when the joint is moved, and for this reason it is necessary for the remedial exercises to be given in a progressive fashion, commencing with a very mild program. The easier way to move an injured shoulder is to allow the arm to hang limply by the side and then flex the body forward from the waist causing the arm to flex itself automatically, being returned to its original position by straightening the trunk. A progression is to rotate the shoulder inwardly and outwardly with the arm dangling forward as before, the next step being to swing the arm gently from side to side, across the body, thus achieving abduction and adduction. Finally, a combination of all these movements by assuming the same trunk-flexed position and gently circling the arm from the shoulder.

The next progression is to lie flat on the floor on one's back, with the arms by the side, then gently slide the arm sideways on the floor until it is outstretched from the shoulder and then on upwards over the head. A further progression is to carry out the exercise in the same manner but include bending and straightening the elbow as the exercise is carried out. In the position shown, all gravity is eliminated and, if the floor be polished, very little friction is encountered. The next progression to this position is to raise the trunk until a half-sitting position is assumed, using a polished board instead of the floor. The same exercises are carried out. Finally, the patient is sitting upright and a normal shoulder movement is attempted. To add to the difficulty of all these exercises, which is, of course, merely a further progression, the length of the lever arm should be increased by holding a stave or short stick in the hand of the moving arm.

The muscles of the upper arm, the triceps and biceps, are sometimes strained, a diagnosis obtained by telling the patient to work the muscles against a light degree of resistance, the site of injury being indicated by pain when the muscle is worked against this resistance. The treatment of these strains takes the same form as indicated elsewhere for strained muscles: application of a firm pressure bandage initially to control the swelling and blood clot formation, light exercises for twenty-four to thirty-six hours, after which heat, massage and progressive remedial exercises may be given.

There is a painful condition of the elbow joint, known as "tennis elbow" peculiar to players of racquet games, javelin throwers and golfers. Caused by a sudden jerk of the arm when making a backhand stroke at tennis, for example, it consists of about four types of injury to the muscles working on the elbow joint. It can also be caused by the athlete suddenly using a racquet or javelin either lighter or heavier than that to which he is accustomed. This misnamed condition can also be acquired in a variety of everyday ways completely unconnected with tennis racquets and javelins. Some of these causes may well prevail in the world of dancing. Many cases begin as a strain, the patient having a circulating poison within his body from an infected tooth, for example, which may settle in the origin of the extensor muscles of the forearm at the outside of the elbow joint, this being rather a weak spot. Diagnosis is made by flexing the wrist and then strengthening the elbow, pain being caused at a small area on the outside of the elbow joint and sometimes running down the belly of the extensor muscles on the front and outer side of the forearm. The pain comes on when anything is gripped tightly in the hand, extension of the elbow and supination of the hand being difficult and painful.

If this condition is left untreated it will generally clear up in about a year, and seldom returns even if the actions originally responsible are again undertaken. The treatment usually boils down to manipulation for those types with painful movement or limitation of movement, while those types with an exquisitely painful spot on the outside of the elbow often need rest, with possible injection of an anaesthetic. Physical treatment should always be given a trial as it often clears up the condition; manipulation is often reserved for those types which are obstinate or where recovery is urgent. Needless to say, all forms of treatment to this condition are of a somewhat specialized nature and should only be undertaken by a qualified and experienced person.

A sprain of the wrist joint is treated in the same fashion as other sprains: by means of the immediate application of cold compresses, followed by adhesive strapping support, later heat, massage and strengthening exercises. In this connection, it should be a rule that no such injury as "sprained wrist" exists until it has been proved by x-ray that the more serious injury of a fracture of the carpal scaphoid bone does not exist. This is one of the most frequent injuries to the wrist joint, and one of the most overlooked because of the difficulty frequently encountered in detecting the injury even by x-rays. The signs of the injury are tenderness and swelling over the bone at the base of the thumb, painful and limited movement of the wrist and thumb particularly when carrying the hand backwards (extension of the wrist) and carrying it sideways to the thumb side. A fractured scaphoid is an injury with a high nuisance value because it is necessary to have the forearm and the lower half of the hand encased in a plaster cast for a period of from three to six months. This is because the bone has a poor blood supply and bony union is extremely slow. During the period that the limb is in plaster, it is essential that regular thumb and finger exercises are carried out, thus maintaining the strength and mobility of these structures and of the muscles of the forearm.

Following injury to the fingers the danger is that the fingers will become stiff and painful. It is essential that great care is taken to ensure a correct balance between rest and exercise; excessive swelling is a sign that movement has been too vigorous and that the part should be rested from gripping, etc. Sprains and strains of the joints of the fingers require mainly exercise, aided by the relaxation afforded by the application of heat. It is therefore a sound idea to have the fingers exercised in a bowl of hot water, or hot wax, and for the patient to carry with him, in his pocket, a small rubber ball on which he is constantly gripping and pressing.

A contusion to the finger will frequently cause the nail to become blackened and to have blood secreted below it. This may be relieved by carefully drilling the nail with a sharp instrument, taking care that the tool is adequately sterilized first, and as the head of blood commences to well out of the bored hole a small drop of peroxide will aid the flow. Lacerations and abrasions to the hand and fingers should be cleaned and dressed in an aseptic fashion, and kept covered until such time as the wound is obviously healing cleanly.

It is necessary to issue a word of warning concerning a condition with the frightening name of Volkmann's Ischaemic Contracture. This is caused by a partial and temporary stoppage of both arterial and venous circulation, frequently in the forearm, causing degeneration of the muscles and swelling of the tissues. It is caused by pressure on the vessels by splints, plaster or tight bandages, or by injury to the arteries and veins in the area. The results are initially severe and increasing pain, with swelling and discoloration of the hand and fingers, and serious damage can be done in a very short time. A "claw-hand" appears in twenty-four hours and, ultimately if the pressure is not relieved, there is necrosis (death) of the skin and muscles on the front of the arm below the elbow. It is therefore of the utmost importance to ensure that no bandaging is too tight when applied to the lower arm or leg, and the patient must be warned as to safety measure if discomfort occurs for this reason.

# PART IV
# TREATMENT OF INJURIES

# 19

# The Treatment of Sprains

A sprain can truly be said to be one of the most common injuries of everyday life. Few people, whatever their age, can say that they have never had a sprain of one or more joints during their school days, sports career, or in later life when their gait might not be quite so sure. The sprain is an injury that can be avoided by some foresight, and can be rapidly cured, never to return providing that certain vital measures are instituted.

The definition of a true sprain can be said to be the partial or complete tear of one or more ligaments forming a joint or it can be merely a stretching of the ligaments concerned. The cause of the injury is usually a sudden twist or wrench of the bones forming the joint. In the case of a true sprain, it can be said that there will be spontaneous recovery in about three to five weeks, this being the case it can be seen that the principal aim is to accelerate this period of recovery or to keep the dancer active during the period of recovery.

It is not difficult to diagnose a sprain if seen within a short time of its occurrence. It is then possible to locate the site of maximum tenderness accurately over a ligament and not over bone. The situation is very different, however, if a long period of time, such as three or four days, has elapsed before the sprain is seen. By then the joint has become tender and swollen over a large area, and it is difficult to localize the injury to any one ligament.

The most sprained joint of the body is undoubtedly the ankle, the external ligament of that joint being frequently hurt. The movement causing this injury is a turning under of the outer border of the foot, at the same time the front of the foot is doubled under itself. This causes the ligaments stretching in three separate bands from the lower end of the fibula to the outside of the calcaneus and the astragalus bones of the foot, to be stretched or torn. The most forward of the three bands of this ligament is, in its turn, the more frequently injured.

If such an ankle sprain should occur when the unfortunate recipient is away from civilization, on a skiing or hiking tour for instance, the boot should not be removed to see what has happened, as this will allow immediate swelling to occur in an alarming fashion. Alpine troops of the French and Italian armies know that such an injury incurred during training will clear up within three days if the patient keeps the ankle in use, without moving the boot from the foot. These men are issued with a long strap known as a "Coindreau strap" which is used in the event of such an emergency, being secured around the ankle above the joint and brought down and around the foot, from the inside to the outside border. It is then pulled tight so that it takes the strain off the ligament on the outside of the ankle, giving it the necessary support it requires.

The pattern of injury in the case of a sprain can be explained in four stages: firstly, the tearing of the actual tissue and the resulting hemorrhage; secondly the formation of a blood clot (hematoma) ; thirdly, the dispersal of the hematoma by absorption into the blood stream and lastly, healing of the tear by means of the laying down of fibrous tissue.

The treatment of a sprain should ideally commence from the moment the injury is sustained, combining the immediate application of local pressure to the injured site with an early resumption of activity. The application of local pressure within a few minutes of injury is necessary to prevent the accumulation of a large hematoma. The importance of this procedure lies in the fact that the length of time for which the patient is out of action when suffering from a sprain is directly proportional to the size of the hematoma that has to be dispersed.

Cold compresses or cold running water are applied to the injured joint for about twenty to thirty minutes, to aid in controlling the local hemorrhage. Then the ankle joint should be padded with cotton wool, or packed with shaped pieces of sponge rubber, over the top of which a strapping of adhesive elastic tape or crepe bandage is applied. This strapping must be applied in such a fashion as to give support to the injured structure, the foot being held in this position and the strapping applied tightly to retain it.

Early movement is important, but must be of a nonweight-bearing nature, the foot being rhythmicaly flexed and extended periodically, while in a supported position. The strapping mentioned above will restrict movement in the plane that caused the original injury while allowing adequate movement in other directions.

This semi-rest period, combined with nonweight-bearing exercises continues for forty-eight hours, and is then followed by the measures necessary to disperse the accumulated fluid and to restore healthy tissue in the repair of the torn ligament. The dispersal of the fluid is attempted by heat and massage, the heat being given by means of an infra-red lamp, hot towels, etc., while the massage must obviously be directed upwards toward the trunk in accordance with the normal drainage of the limb. It aids to have the limb raised in some form of elevation, with support under the knee by means of a cushion or pillow placed under the heel, thus assisting in the drainage. The supporting strapping is continued although not of such an elaborate nature. More active types of exercises can be given together with supervised weight-bearing, this part of the treatment being progressively increased as the condition improves.

Sprains constitute a recurrent source of danger, in that the torn ligament represents a weak point for a very long time after the original injury has cleared up. For this reason it is preferable that a dancer not be allowed to resume activity following a sprained joint without a strong supporting strapping on the joint in question. This should be carried out with adhesive tape and should follow the same supporting principles that apply when using the compression bandage in the early stages of treatment.

Before leaving sprains of the ankle joint, it would be well to describe the signs and symptoms of the injury, although they are probably well known to all persons. There is momentary pain of a "lightning" character which may radiate up the leg. At the same time the muscles controlling the joint go into a spasm and the abnormal position of the foot and ankle, causing the sprain, is corrected. The patient is usually able to walk after the injury has taken place although probably with a limp, but before many minutes have passed, weight-bearing will cause acute pain of a sickening nature. The ankle swells almost visibly at a very fast rate, and walking becomes increasingly difficult.

The wrist is another joint that is frequently sprained, usually by forcing the hand either backwards or forwards at the moment of injury. This frequently occurs when one falls onto the palm or back of the hand. It is safest to treat such an injury as though it were a fractured scaphoid bone and have it x-rayed, this injury being extremely difficult to diagnose and frequently is overlooked by being called a sprain. The thumb or fingers can be sprained quite easily and form painful and disabling injuries that will remain a nuisance for a considerable period unless accurately treated. Some form of support and fixation is required, preceded by bathing in cold water; this can take the form of adhesive elastic strapping which will give elastic support with some restriction of extreme movements but not complete immobilization.

A complication of the sprained ankle is that of the "chip" fracture, a condition in which the force tearing the ligament also causes a flake of bone to tear away from the ligamentous attachment on the fibula, tibia or tarsal bones of the foot. These cases are treated in much the same fashion as a true sprain, but will take approximately twice the length of time to clear up sufficiently to enable the patient to resume her activity.

# 20

# The Treatment of Strains

The injury sustained in physical activity that is known as the "pulled" muscle is in reality a strained muscle, and constitutes a serious painful condition. It is usually produced by a sudden uneven contraction of muscle, due to lack of coordination and balance of the group of muscles concerned in a specific movement. The actual "pull" consists of a strain, tear or even a complete rupture of a muscle or its tendon; the tissue is actually torn. Possibly only a very few fibers are concerned, although a bad strain will include not only a large number of fibers but also the muscle sheath itself. The rupture can occur at any point in the muscle, either at the origin or insertion of the muscle or in its fleshy belly.

The signs and symptoms of the muscle strain are those of acute pain in the area of the injury, with an immediate and almost complete loss of function of the muscle involved. As a result of the rupture there is injury to the minute blood vessels in the area, resulting in a hemorrhage within the substance of the muscle, leading to the formation of a blood clot (hematoma). The dispersal of this hematoma is the key to the whole healing process, the larger the hematoma the longer the period of absorption, and subsequently the greater the period of disability. The size of the hematoma is controlled by the initial treatment given when the strain occurs; later the clot is able to be softened by means of physiotherapy and dispersed into the blood stream. Finally, the actual muscle fibers are repaired by the laying down of elastic, fibrous tissue which replaces the inevitable scar tissue.

The muscle groups most commonly strained are as follows:

(a) The hamstrings, at the back of the thigh which flex the knee.

(b) The quadriceps, on the front of the thigh, which extend the knee.

(c) The posterior tibial group or calf muscles, which pull the heel upwards.

(d) The biceps muscle of the upper arm, which flexes the elbow and the shoulder joint.

(e) The supraspinatus muscle, on the top of the shoulder, which aids in lifting the arm from the side of the body.

The injury will be very localized, being checked by testing the function of the muscle groups with both free movement and with resisted movement, with slight resistance being applied. Localized tenderness and swelling are invariably present.

Reasons for muscles straining can be classified under three main headings: lack of warming-up, failure to put a muscle group through its fullest range of movement during practice and, thirdly, septic foci. Warming-up is considered to be of such importance that it is covered in a separate chapter of this book.

During the course of their activities, dancers do not always use vital muscle groups in their fullest range, from their most contracted to their most extended position. Subsequently, when a muscle is suddenly stretched to its fullest extent under conditions of stress, it gives way and a "pull" results. A thorough limbering-up routine will give these muscle groups the suppleness they require to fight off strains.

The third reason, that of a septic foci, is a very common one, but a factor little considered when dealing with injuries. If a dancer has about her body some source of poison, such as decayed teeth, bad tonsils or adenoids, she has a distributing center for poisons to radiate throughout her entire body. This establishes a weak link in the muscle fortifications, causing the weakest point in the muscle to give way when placed to strain and stress.

The treatment of muscle strains follows a strict sequence: firstly the athlete is withdrawn from activity, an essential measure, otherwise a minor tear can be aggravated into a major lesion. To enable an artiste to perform free of pain the injection of anaesthetic into the area might be considered. Such a procedure is both dangerous and unlikely to succeed. In a badly damaged muscle, one that is grossly torn, this masking of the pain—nature's danger signal—could lead to it becoming completely ruptured because of the patient's inability to feel the pain resulting from aggravation of the injury. There may well be a place in the treatment of injuries for such treatment but this is not it!

Initially, cold compresses are applied to the area of injury, thus controlling the internal bleeding, for a period of about fifteen to twenty minutes. But in the case of an obviously bad strain it is better to omit this feature and go straight ahead with the application of a pressure bandage. This is a supporting, controlling bandage reaching from about nine inches above the injury to the same distance below it, and consisting of alternate layers of cotton wool and crepe bandage, the whole forming a bulky packing which controls the swelling and fluid. This bandage is worn for the next thirty-six hours, during which time the patient rests the injury, while exercising in a nonweight-bearing fashion. This type of exercise consists of contracting the muscles without actually moving the joints on which they work, or by means of light, rhythmic exercises. This procedure ensures that the muscles retain tone and volume, at the same time carrying out a form of automatic massage, by means of their alternate contraction and relaxation against the elastic pressure of the bandage, thus exerting a pumping action aiding in the dispersal of the accumulated fluid.

It is essential that no form of heat or massage is permitted during this thirty-six hours' period to the site of injury. Torn muscle bleeds and the effect of heat or massage is to increase the local circulation, thus enhancing this bleeding, causing a much larger hematoma to form, with far greater trouble in its disposal. At the end of the thirty-six hours' period proper treatment can begin, consisting of gentle massage, preceded by some form of heat, and concluded by a scheme of exercises progressively designed to build up the muscle group and restore strength. The heat and massage are required to disperse the fluids which are painfully stretching the tissues around the injured part, although the immediate measures should have restricted them to a minimum. This part of the treatment is progressively increased so that it is breaking down and softening the hematoma and aiding in its dispersal. The exercises are gradually replaced by a more active form of activity, taking care all the time that the muscle concerned is not unduly stretched, until full activity can be resumed. It will usually be found that weight-bearing exercises can be started on about the tenth day following the injury, and the condition should be cleared up sufficiently within three to four weeks to resume training. However, dogmatism in any form of medicine is the height of optimism and the disability period depends upon numerous factors, the co-ordination or otherwise of which can shorten or lengthen the time for which the patient is out of action.

It is stated by some medical authorities that there is inevitably permanently weakened function of a muscle following a "pull." The case put forward is that repair takes place in such a fashion that normal tissue is replaced by inelastic scar tissue, which presumably prevents the muscle from ever regaining its former strength. This being the case, if it is to be accepted, prevention is obviously better than cure, because few active dancers will go through their career without some form of muscular strain, either minor or severe. Yet another school of thought maintains that regular, competent massage given throughout the rehabilitation period will replace the inelastic scar tissue by healthy tissue because of the greatly improved local circulation brought about by the massage.

# 21

# The Treatment of Contusions

Violent and energetic activities carry with them the risk of taking knocks, either by falling, colliding with another person or by hitting against hard objects. In this way is caused the contusion—a blow that does not break the skin but causes a bruise.

The crushing of the soft tissues of the body by a violent external force, without causing a break in the continuity of the skin, will cause certain visible signs. There will be obvious pain on movement, and through outside pressure; there will be discoloration ranging from yellow to black, and there will almost invariably be swelling. In the case of those tissues of the body that are lax or loose, such as the eyelids or the scrotum, the discoloration will be very much more marked, as is seen when a "black eye" is sustained.

The normal, uncomplicated bruise will rarely become worse after the first twenty-four hours or so. It will progressively improve with adequate treatment and exercise. It can be termed an "immediate" injury, because its effects are felt almost at once, with the exception of the knock that passes unnoticed when the dancer is hot and moving during the course of a performance, but stiffens up rapidly when she pauses. Thus it can be said that the first principle of treatment with anything other than a really severe contusion is for the person to continue moving about as much as possible if she wishes to continue her activity.

The immediate treatment, therefore, is to keep the part warm by means of movement, plus the artificial aid of massage with capsicum vaseline (chili paste) which will give a general sensation of warmth and will greatly aid in relieving the pain. Different measures, however, must prevail when a serious knock is sustained, when a really hard, violent force strikes the thigh, for example, causing what is known in America as a "charley-horse." Initially, there is bleeding within the tissue substance at the site of injury; this internal hemorrhage is caused by the rupture of many minute blood vessels within the injured area, due to the crushing effect of the blow. Secondly, the internal bleeding eventually forms a blood clot (hematoma) within the substance of the tissues, the eventual dispersal of this clot causing the marked bruising and discoloration that often appears well below the site of the injury.

The crux of the treatment of a contusion lies in the rapid dispersal of this blood clot, which has to be "broken up" so that it can be absorbed into the normal blood stream and so taken away from the inflamed and painful area. It is obvious that the smaller the clot, the less time it will take to be dispersed—hence one's first aim of treatment is to ensure that the size of the clot is controlled as early as possible. This is done by means of the application of cold and the use of pressure bandage. It is not always possible to apply cold compresses or ice as soon as the injury occurs, but there is no reason for the absence of some form of pressure bandage at once. It can take the form of the usual alternate layers of bandage and cotton wool, if it is not intended for the dancer to remain on the stage or it can be 'formed of firm strapping with elastic adhesive bandage. The benefit of this latter form of bandage, coupled with its enabling the artiste to continue dancing, is that the elastic pressure of the strapping, together with the alternate relaxation and contraction of the muscles concerned, cause a form of "auto-massage" which aids in dispersing the inevitable outpouring of fluids within the tissues.

Immediately it is possible, apply ice, ice water, cold compresses or pads soaked in ether-meth. or surgical spirit to the injured area. Continue this for about one-half hour, then apply a pressure bandage and instruct the injured person gently to brace (alternate contract and relax) her muscles against the pressure of the bandage, with the limb in an elevated and resting position.

This situation prevails for twenty-four hours, after which steps must be taken to aid the absorption of the blood clot, and the laying down of tissue to replace any that has been severed or displaced by the force of the blow. This is done by means of heat and massage, together with sensible nonweight-bearing mobilizing exercises at first, progressing onwards to stronger and more active exercises as the condition improves. At first, the area may be found to be too tender to permit massage, in which case the patient should be instructed to sit on the side of a bath with a towel wrapped around the injured part, and pour hot water over the towel. The system is for three jugs of hot water to be used then one jug of cold water and so on, for about twenty minutes. After that, the limb will be found to be in a supple and fairly mobile condition, thus permitting exercises of a remedial nature. Finish up by applying the pressure bandage for the first few days, as injured tissue always feels more comfortable when it is supported. Massage should be of a loosening nature, and should not necessarily be extremely painful. It is essential, however, throughout the period of treatment that the artiste is encouraged to move the part and to carry out home exercises and hot towels; contusions will almost always improve spontaneously and this form of home treatment can do nothing but good.

The one exception to this program of treatment for a contusion is when the complication of myositis ossificans traumatica or ossifying hematoma occurs. This is described more fully in the chapter on the more serious injuries, but it should be said again here that the above treatment as laid down will greatly worsen any contusion that has a tendency to calcify, and a close watch should be kept for the signs and symptoms of this condition, as laid down in the later chapter.

A contusion to a joint will invariably cause an outpouring of fluid within the joint, which arises from the lining membrane of the joint known as the synovial membrane, and the condition is known as synovitis. The immediate treatment is the application of a firm pressure bandage, using either cotton wool and bandages or shaped pieces of sponge rubber placed around the joint where necessary and held in position with a firm bandage. The later treatment is largely one of exercise, with heat and massage if necessary. Hot towels are useful in dispersing fluid, but the primary treatment should be directed toward clearing up the original injury that caused the outpouring of fluid.

At various parts of the body nerves are exposed to external violence, such an area being the head or top of the fibula bone which runs down the outside of the lower leg. At this spot, the external popliteal nerve runs around the head of the bone and is very vulnerable. Any blow struck on such an exposed part will cause pain to run down the course of the nerve and will affect the area of the body supplied by that nerve, the total effect lasting for a period which may range from seconds to hours. There will frequently be a temporary paralysis of the muscles controlled by the injured nerve, and the sensation of "pins and needles" will be experienced in the area. It is important to treat the psychological side of this type of injury, because the artiste invariably tends to panic when she discovers the temporary paralysis, consequently she has to be reassured. The treatment is mild heat application and rest, with NO massage over the injured area. When activity is resumed the part can be protected against further injury by means of adhesive felt or sponge rubber padding.

Contusions to bone are obstinate conditions to clear up. Every bone is covered in its entirety with a thin film of protective cartilage known as the periosteum, and once bruised it is a sore spot for a considerable period. The tenderness seems as though it has to "wear out" of of the bone, and makes itself felt for a long time. A very frequent area suffering from this type of injury is that of the sole of the foot, caused by the artiste jumping on a hard surface from a height or upon a stone when running. The subsequent deep and painful bruising of the thick tissue on the sole of the foot is treated by means of some form of deep heating, ideally short-wave diathermy. Hot water can be used as a substitute followed by deep fingertip friction-type massage. It is important further to protect the injured area from damage by means of padding with adhesive felt or sponge rubber.

# 22

# The Treatment of Lacerations and Abrasions

It can be assumed with every degree of certainty that at some time or other almost everyone who participates in active physical exercise will receive a laceration or an abrasion. This skin wound will usually be irregularly torn and bruised through contact of a hard object.

These wounds can usually be classified under four headings:

    (1) Incised wounds
    (2) Lacerated wounds.
    (3) Punctured wounds.
    (4) Contused wounds.

The incised wound has sharp, well-defined edges, caused by a blow on tightly stretched skin. The edges remain closed but will gape when the part is moved. There will usually be profuse bleeding, as blood vessels have been cut. This type of injury will often require suturing (stitching) by a doctor, and providing it is initially cleaned in a satisfactory fashion, it should heal in five to seven days without scarring.

The lacerated wound is a jagged, irregular affair, with bruised edges such as might be caused by the impact of an object such as a cricket ball. The mildest type of laceration is the most common of injuries, the abrasion or graze. This type of injury rarely bleeds very much, heals slowly and leaves unpleasant scarring. It also presents a frequent risk of infection.

The puncture wound is that caused by a spike or nail, and has a small entrance but with a large, hidden interior usually containing dirt. Fort this reason, it is frequently necessary for the doctor to carry out what is known as a debridement, or an enlarging operation with his intruments. This exposes the interior of the wound for the necessary cleansing treatment.

A contused wound is any wound associated with bruising, and is therefore frequently classified under the heading of incised or lacerated.

The treatment of lacerations and abrasions must always be carried out under conditions of the utmost sterility, the instruments used should have initially been boiled for twenty minutes and brought straight from the water to the wound that is to be treated. Assemble all the materials required on a clean towel—bowls, antiseptics, warm water, dressings, forceps, scissors, etc. As each cotton wool swab is used, it should be placed in a separate container as it is no longer free from infection. If it is possible, all swabs should be used by holding in a previously sterilized pair of forceps. Clean the wound from the center outwards, thus taking dirt from the center of the wound to its edges. Use each swab in this way once only, and finish up by cleaning the surrounding skin.

The cleansing solution can either be a solution composed of one part of dettol to twenty parts of warm water, diluted eusol, or a specific wound cleanser such as cetavlon. To dress the wound, use a pad of gauze or white lint, with an emulsion of acriflavine, which will prevent the dressing from adhering to the wound and cause a scab to form over it. The usual bandage, or adhesive plaster dressing can then be applied.

If the wound required stitching, clean in a similar fashion and then apply a soft pad of lint or gauze to the wound until the arrival of the doctor who will stitch the laceration. After this operation is completed, there are two principal types of dressings which may be applied. A pad of lint dressing covered by a piece of cotton wool if the patient is to be sent home. This form of pressure bandage will aid in preventing swelling and will also make the patient comfortable. Should it be necessary for the injured person to return to the stage, a different type of dressing is required. This is formed by laminating several separate thicknesses of gauze by means of collodion, or liquid skin. This forms a firm, adherent dressing which will remain in place for the remainder of the performance.

A graze or abrasion that has dirt contained within it will have to be cleaned by means of warm water and soap, and gentle scrubbing with a nail brush. After this, the usual dressings are applied.

A wound that is going to require stitching should never have any sort of colored antiseptic, such as acriflavine or gentian violet, applied before the actual stitching, otherwise it will require cleansing again before the actual operation.

When a man gets hurt outdoors, and his wound is of such a nature that the skin is broken, there always will be present great danger of infection through dirt entering the wound, or in some cases because of fertilizer used on the area. If the wound is badly impregnated with mud and dirt it is a safe measure to have the person inoculated with anti-tetanus serum, but it must be ensured that this injection is not given at less than two-yearly intervals otherwise a very adverse reaction is sometimes experienced.

The more severe lacerations will require some form of stitching or clipping, thus forming a wound with its edges held together, a situation which facilitates healing without extensive scarring. The stitches or sutures used are of two types—absorbable and non-absorbable. The former are made from catgut, kangaroo tendon, etc., and are used for deep structures and internal operations. The non-absorbable type are manufactured from silkworm gut, horsehair, linen thread and silk, and are used for the more superficial regions, such as the face and head. The needles used are straight, half-circle, three-eighth circle or J-shaped, and can be round-bodied or cutting type. The round-bodied are used for muscles and viscera, while the cutting-type needles are used for skin and tendons. The various methods of stitching can be summarized under the headings of continuous, interrupted or tied, interlocking or mattress. There are also two or three types of minute spring clips, which can be applied to hold the wound edges together, but these clips are never used on the face for fear of scarring.

Obviously, a wound must be perfectly clean before it can be stitched. Firstly, the wound must be carefully cleaned with one of the solutions already mentioned— mild dettol, eusol or cetavlon. The cotton wool swab should be held in the sterilized forceps and the solution applied so that the wound is cleaned from the center to its edges, and never in the reverse fashion so that dirt is brushed from the surrounding skin into the wound. As already warned, never use any form of antiseptic that will dye the area of the wound. Some doctors will pack the wound with penicillin styptic powder before stitching, thus aiding in halting the inevitable bleeding. After the wound has been stitched, a clean, dry dressing is applied, backed by a pad of cotton wool, thus forming a comfortable dressing that will control any swelling.

The collodion dressing already described should be used if it is desired to return the artiste to the stage, as this gives a protective layer over the wound when dry and there is more than a reasonable chance of the dressing remaining in place despite the most strenuous activity.

Stitches are usually removed within five to seven days. This is done by the doctor or a nurse, who, using a pair of sterilized forceps and scissors will hold and cut each stitch as near to the skin as possible, drawing the longer end gently free from the now enclosed wound edges.

# 23

# The Treatment of Skin Infections

It can truly be said that the minor injury of today can rapidly turn into the major injury of tomorrow. This applies particularly to infections of the skin, which are rarely given the consideration that they merit. It does not seem to be realized that a dancer can miss a performance through a painful skin condition, such as sunburn, just as easily as through a pulled muscle. It is not always possible to prevent strains, sprains, contusions, etc., but it is frequently possible to carry out preliminary measures and precautions that will keep the dancer safe from the more common skin infections.

There are certain common skin infections which are easy to acquire, difficult to disperse and which will spread through the studio like a prairie fire. Before passing on to them and their signs and symptoms, it is necessary for an idea to be given of the structure and functions of the skin.

The functions of the skin are:

(1) To act as a protective covering.

(2) As an organ of secretion via the sweat glands.

(3) The lubrication of the outer covering of the body, through the sebaceous glands contained within the skin, which give off sebum, the sub-

210

stance which lubricates the skin. The skin is supplied with blood vessels, nerves, and has an outer horny layer, the nails forming a modification of this horny layer, known as keratin. This outer layer is protected from external irritants by the sweat and sebum.

In some cases there is a surplus of sebum, this lubricant of the skin, which causes the skin to become excessively oily. This results in conditions such as acne and seborrhoea. The hairs possess roots within the skin, which are known as follicles. The masseur who uses some types of oil when massaging, or who fails to use any sort of lubricant whatsoever so that his hands "pull" as he massages, will frequently cause the hairs to be forcibly pulled from their roots. The oil or other foreign matter enters the minute holes that are thus left in the skin, causing them to become blocked, infection is caused and results in a rash-like condition known as folliculitis.

One of the most common physical reactions encountered is that of the common blister, a minor blight suffered by every dancer at some time or other during her career. Caused by ill-fitting shoes,* darned or holed socks, pressure on a soft part of the feet, etc., they are extremely tender and can be crippling temporarily. The main treatment is that of prevention, which is much better than cure, and blisters can be averted by the use of various measures already described.

Inflammation of the skin, known as dermatitis, can be caused by either physical or infective means. The physical reason is by far the most common and is due to

---

* Blisters in dancers are nearly always caused by tight shoes. They have to be this way, particularly for the boys or they will not stay on.

an excess of heat or cold, chemicals, sun's rays, x-rays, friction or pressure of some kind, etc. The type resulting from infection is caused by bacteria, fungi or parasites. Impetigo is very contagious; it is recognized by large, crusted areas on the face, neck and ears. As already mentioned, it is highly contagious and therefore can be spread through a group by contact extremely easily. It is important not to use any of the sulphonamide group of drugs when treating this condition, the best treatment being calamine, with a mild antiseptic, or 1 to 4,000 perchloride of mercury.

Boils are caused by germs, known as staphylococci, which are normally found in large numbers on the skin. It would seem, therefore, that boils are caused by some breakdown in the local skin defence mechanism, which permits these ever-present germs to have a harmful effect. As has already been explained, large numbers of boils are caused through the blocking of the hair roots, or follicles. In the case of dancers, the skin breakdown is often caused through friction of the clothing, such as wet tights rubbing the inside of the thighs, or the friction caused by clothes dampened by sweat.

The prevention of boils can be attempted by first raising the general standard of health, then by hardening the skin with spirit, and by changing the clothing frequently. The treatment of a small boil can be attempted by covering it with a small piece of adhesive elastic plaster and leaving it alone. The larger boil can be treated by having dressings of magnesium sulphate placed upon it, or if greater drawing powers are required, a rather drastic but highly effective method is to apply a small kaolin poultice over the top of a magnesium sulphate dressing. A boil can also be treated by means of hot fomentations made from Milton or eusol, placed upon the boil every four hours. The boil should be covered with a dry dressing in between fomentations. The injection of penicillin by the doctor will speedily clear up a boil, and will also prevent others occurring, it being usual to give three injections on three successive days.

Sunburn is a very painful and easily acquired condition. It can be prevented by placing a screen on the skin of ointment containing ten percent para-aminobenzoic acid in a cold cream base. If the skin has already been burned, it can be treated by means of application of calamine lotion, and if it is an extremely severe burn, cold compresses should be applied and the patient rested in a darkened room.

In most communities, one or more members will be discovered who are allergic to the application of adhesive plaster. The use of this form of dressing on such a person may cause dermatitis over the area that has been covered by the plaster. In some people who are ultrasensitive, it is not even possible to apply plaster over a bandage, as even with such precautions a rash will be caused exactly where the plaster has covered.

To prevent such an irritation the skin should be first shaved cleanly before the application of the plaster, then the area should be painted with friars balsam (tincture benzoin). This causes the skin to be protected and the plaster to adhere more firmly, although allowing it to be removed freely. When the plaster is eventually removed, the skin over which it has been affixed should be cleaned with spirit and then covered with a film of calamine lotion or talcum powder. To remove the plaster take a bath still wearing it, the hot water greatly aids in loosening the plaster and facilitates its easy removal. Another method of removal is to ease it off, using spirit to neutralize the adhesive as the plaster is gently lifted. A third effective, but drastic, method, is to tell the patient to "hold tight" and rapidly rip the plaster from the limb in one swift movement—often it is found that it is best to be cruel to be kind.

To obviate all the trouble of removal it is sometimes possible to apply the plaster in a reversed fashion, that is, with the sticky side uppermost, the adhesive can be neutralized by means of rubbing cotton wool over it or using talcum powder.

# 24

# The Treatment of Miscellaneous Injuries

All the injuries of active exercise and the many factors arising from them cannot be classified neatly into specific sections and paragraphs. Many occasions will arise when the teacher will be confronted with a problem, sometimes major and more frequently minor, the solution of which will not at first be apparent nor will she be able readily to ascertain sources of information sufficient to answer her questions.

The usual medical advice given to the unfortunate athlete or dancer with some form of injury includes invariably the word "rest." Undoubtedly this is a safe and conservative method of dealing with an injury, but rarely will it clear up the condition and inevitably rest will cause the victim to lose many weeks of activity and to lapse into a state of comparative weakness. The injured person is frequently in a quandary as to whether she should rest an injury or exercise it. On the face of it, one would consider that the practice of lying-up or rest with a painful knock, one that limits movements and causes discomfort, to be a reasonable procedure. This line of reasoning is incorrect, however, and it is dangerous and completely wrong to rest entirely the type of acute injury sustained in physical activity.

In the year 1867, a very famous surgeon of his day

was Sir James Paget, who stated: "Too long rest is by far the most frequent cause of delayed recovery to joints and to joints that are kept at rest because of injury to muscles working on them." Although Sir James had no hesitation in condemning the then prevalent practice of complete rest, it is regretted that the doctors of his day took little notice of the internationally renowned surgeon. It is similarly regretted that the majority of doctors practicing today exhibit an identical state of indifference.

Generally speaking, it can be said that the only type of condition arising from an injury sustained in active exercise that requires complete rest is one that is infected—a bacterial condition. Complete rest is directly responsible for a considerable amount of later trouble, following an injury, due to the formation of adhesions. An adhesion is a limiting, contracted band or area of scar tissue due to the formation of inflammatory products in the injured area during periods of inactivity. The injured dancer should be advised to exercise the injury gently, keeping within the bounds of tolerable pain, and watching for any marked aggravation of the injury which will denote excessive exercise due to overenthusiasm. Should it be the legs that are affected, the exercises should be of a nonweight-bearing nature, that is, exercises performed in a sitting or lying position so that no actual body weight is transmitted to the legs. Possibly the most simple exercise of this type is a static muscular contraction, such as occurs when the muscles on the front of the thighs, the quadriceps, are braced. Another simple form of nonweight-bearing exercise consists of elementary flexion and extension (bending and stretching) of the knees or ankles with the legs outstretched on a bed or couch. Ideally, such forms of exercise should be supervised by a qualified and experienced person, but if this is not possible, the teacher should carefully teach the table of exercises to the patient, demonstrating initially on the sound, uninjured limb.

Rare is the teacher who has never been approached by a stiffly-moving, miserable pupil complaining bitterly of muscular stiffness, usually at the commencement of the season. This very prevalent complaint can just about be classified under the heading of a sports injury, because muscular stiffness can materially affect the performance of the athlete or dancer, even possibly preventing them from turning out. There appears to be no satisfactory explanation for the onset of stiffness, nor is it known why its effects are felt some hours after exercise.

It is known that muscle fibers swell after strenuous or prolonged activity, thus forming a larger number of the minute particles, known as molecules, that collectively go to form material substances such as muscular tissue. The increased number of molecules formed attract water, in the form of body fluids, inwards, so that the spaces between the cells, in which the nerves and blood vessels lie, gets smaller. It can be seen therefore, that these nerve fibers are compressed, giving rise to painful sensations during movement as the muscle fibers return to their normal size during later recovery.

Stiffness will follow an unusual type of exercise, however, although the person concerned may be in an excellent state of fitness, and when fatigue has not necessarily been experienced. This may result from undue stretching of muscles, making them oversensitive, so that subsequent slight movements cause an abnormal or exaggerated reaction, known as "stretch reflex." It is also possible that a small proportion of muscle fibers are actually torn or ruptured, but give rise to pain only when they begin to heal.

It is possible to prevent stiffness by means of easy progression in the severity of the exercises used in early training days. After these preliminary training sessions, the pupil should have a hot bath, with a cupful of ordinary soda added. There should be no hanging about after activity, so that the dancer becomes chilled. Gentle massage given after a particularly strenuous training session will aid in preventing stiffness. Make the second session of training as near to the first as possible—little and often is far superior to one hard lengthy period per week. Should stiffness occur in spite of all these precautions, give some form of heat by means of a lamp, hot baths, or towels, followed by massage, and concluding with gentle exercise movements growing progressively more strenuous. If the dancer warms up well before commencing her exercises, she will find that she tends not to stiffen as much as previously. Though more exhausting it is more beneficial for a dancer to work during hot weather when she can warm up quicker and can work harder with less chance of injury.

The dancer who suffers from cramp will always be with us, but far less frequently if a few simple preliminary steps are taken to prevent it. Invariably caused by loss of salt due to excessive sweating, it can be cured by taking more salt with meals. Should this not suffice, a course of quinine sulphate tablets will usually do the trick. Should cramp occur during an actual performance it should be treated by stretching the affected muscle group, and with gentle massage of a relaxing nature. Young dancers in the early stages of training often suffer from cramp in the feet due to the effort of stretching.

A very frequent mis-diagnosis encountered is that of synovitis. All joints are lined with a spongy membrane from which is given the fluid that "lubricates" the joint, and which is known as the synovial membrane. Almost any injury sustained by a joint will cause this membrane to be damaged, causing an abnormal outpouring of fluid to issue from it. The error in diagnosis lies in the fact that the condition is not an injury in its own right, but a reaction to an injury. The cure therefore lies in treating the underlying injury that causes the membrane to be damaged; until this is cleared up, surplus fluid will continue to swell the joint.

The immediate treatment is to apply a firm pressure bandage, using either alternate layers of cotton wool and a bandage, or shaped pieces of adhesive felt or sponge rubber under a bandage. Later treatment is largely one of exercise, with heat and massage if required.

The dancer is sometimes worried by a painful and rather puzzling swelling in her groin, which invariably comes up suddenly and persists for a few days. This condition is known as adenitis and is caused by the dancer having a wound, such as a blister, on her foot or lower leg, which has become infected. In the groin, as in other parts of the body, are glands, known as lymph glands, which will filter off the poison from this septic wound, whether it be on the foot, knee, or anywhere on the limb. This filtering off of the poison causes the glands to become inflamed and painfully swollen.

The treatment is directed toward clearing up the septic wound so that the swollen glands will again become normal. Three or four injections of penicillin are sometimes required to abort or disperse the infection, and the swelling and pain rapidly vanish.

# 25

# The Treatment of the More Serious Injuries

There are certain relatively serious injuries and conditions sustained on thankfully rare occasions that will occasionally confront the alarmed teacher. In few cases will she be sufficiently experienced or competent to undertake the necessary treatment, but it will be to her advantage to have some degree of familiarity with these more serious injuries. It can truly be said that a little knowledge is a dangerous thing, and it is hoped that the intelligent teacher will learn from experience as to what she should not do and when to leave well enough alone.

The turns and jumps of ballet dancing can, in a confined space be as dangerous to the performers as the body-contact activities of the sports field and deaths have been known to occur as a result of sports injuries. Sixty-six percent of these fatalities result from injuries to the head and neck and their complications. Falling scenery has been known to cause serious head injuries. The most frequent head injury that will be encountered is probably that of concussion, of which there are three types:

Type 1. The mild type, with momentary loss of consciousness.

Type 2. The mild type with no actual loss of consciousness, but the victim is said to be "out on her feet."

Type 3. When the subject is unconscious for a minute or more, leaving in its wake headache, dizziness and partial or complete loss of intellect.

To be perfectly on the safe side, the subject suffering from any one of the above types should be withdrawn from activity, but in actual practice it is only the third type that usually causes the artist to cut short her work. Therefore, when either of the first two types occur, take the usual first aid measure for restoring consciousness, and if the patient seems in reasonable condition, allow her to resume. The third type is far more serious, the patient is cold, covered with a clammy sweat, her breathing is slow, the pupils are contracted. The recovery of consciousness is usually accompanied by nausea and vomiting. The patient must be kept warm, a doctor sent for and all preparations made to send the patient to hospital; before that occurs, however, the patient should be kept prone with her head turned to one side.

In simple cases, the pupils of the eyes are always equal in size, if they are unequal it should be considered as evidence of a more serious condition, such as cerebral compression. To test a doubtful concussion case, the memory should be questioned as amnesia is a symptom. Question her on recent events, ask her the date, etc. Vagueness or hesitation indicates that the subject is suffering from concussion. Another test is that which elicits nystagmus, a sideways, oscillatory movement of the eyeballs, the patient lacking the ability to follow with her eyes a finger passed slowly backwards and forwards before her face.

An extremely serious injury is that of fracture of the skull, which possesses certain recognizable symptoms among which are unconsciousness, shock, discharge of blood or fluid from ears, nose or mouth, bleeding into whites of eyes, vomiting and paralysis of some muscles of the side of the face. It is very uncommon to find all these symptoms in a case, but a fracture of the base of the skull should be suspected if even a small amount of blood is found escaping from the ear, for example. The presence of one or more signs, with or without unconsciousness must be assumed to be due to a fractured skull. The patient must be kept still in a lying position with her head on one side, warmth must be maintained and no drinks given. Immediate hospitalization is essential, and can make the difference between life and death.

One of the most serious injuries is that of a fracture of a bone, an injury that is sometimes extremely difficult to detect. Therefore it is important that the teacher has some idea of the signs and symptoms of a fracture, thus avoiding any of the more serious complications caused by allowing a dancer to aggravate her condition by continuing with such a serious injury. The diagnosis is usually made by means of the history of the occurrence, and by the symptoms and the signs that are present. The injured dancer usually states that she felt "something give way" and there is severe pain and loss of use of the affected limb. There is a general symptom of shock, and the local signs are those of pain which can be lessened by gentle handling. Adequate medical aid must be obtained at once.

It is usual for loss of power to be complete and attempts by the patient to "test" her injured limb should be prevented. The bone will frequently be found to be tender along its course, and deformity will be present; this can best be discovered by comparison with the uninjured limb. There will be irregularity and a sharp edge or a bump will be felt, but the rapid swelling in the area

will tend to mask this sign. Although extremely difficult
to detect, when a lower limb is injured, the fractured leg
will sometimes be found to be shorter than the other leg.
There is very rapid swelling in the area of the break,
which will increase as the bruising becomes more evident.
A grating sound is sometimes heard, known as crepitus.
It is caused by the broken ends of bone moving over each
other. Under no circumstances should the limb be pur-
posely moved to elicit this crepitus, nor should it be tested
for unnatural movement, which is in itself positive evidence of a fracture.

Obviously, the above symptoms are rarely all present
at the same time, and diagnosis can be made on the evidence presented by one or more of them. If there is severe
pain in a limb after a heavy fall or a hard collision, with
bone tenderness and shock, then suspicion of a fracture
is a correct precaution.

It is possible for bones to be fractured, or brought to
the point of fracture, by sudden strong muscular contraction. A gradual build-up of aggravation to a bone and its
muscular attachments can lead to a "stress-fracture" if
the activities causing the trouble are not halted. Such occurrences are not uncommon in the bones of the lower leg
(the tibia and fibula particularly at the start of the season.
The inner border of the shinbone (tibia) will be tender
and ache; this can be caused by jumping with the hips
rotated outwards. Another cause can be a jarring of the
bone through inadequate use of the joints of the feet as
shock absorbers. Either cause can be put down to faulty
technique but fatigue can also be at the bottom of it.

As there is a danger of a spontaneous fracture of the
bone if the trouble is allowed to persist, jumping should
cease until all symptoms have subsided. Sometimes, pain

and tenderness can be felt about two inches above the ankle bone on the outside of the leg. They are caused by jumping and persist for three weeks or so; rest is required. An allied condition is known to the athlete as "shin-splints"—a tearing of some fibers of the calf muscles from the bone through constant movement or jumping on hard surfaces. It is usually met early in the season before the muscles have acquired sufficient strength to fight off injury. The continual, constant jarring causes pain. particularly on movement, in the region of the lower and outer third of the leg.

This condition is most obstinate and slow to clear up, heat and massage frequently appear to irritate the injured area, in which case rest, with nonweight-bearing exercises, has been the treatment of choice. No two cases appear to respond to the same treatment and methods of treatment carried out by the author include the following:

1. Short wave diathermy, with rest and nonweight-bearing exercises.
2. Hot towels, followed by massage of a squeezing nature in which the bulk of the calf muscles are pressed around the tibia and moved around the bone. Exercises and strapping.
3. Rest, with nonweight-bearing exercises and strapping.
4. Massage with hot olive oil, followed by exercises and support with a heavy elastic-weave bandage.

In each case the patient is given a sponge rubber heel to wear inside the heel of every shoe worn during the period of the injury. At the same time she is warned not to change into low-heeled slippers, thus causing more strain on the posterior tibial muscles and their tendon of insertion. The strapping in question is composed of overlapping separate strips of elastic adhesive plaster, bound in a three-quarter circular strapping so that the gastrochemius is squeezed around the posterior surface of the tibia. This strapping will give almost instantaneous relief and materially aids in dispersing the condition, although its effects only last for as long as it is maintained. It is remotely possible to confuse this condition with a crack fracture of the fibula, and if doubt exists radiography should be used to establish the diagnosis.

Another easily acquired injury is the "stress" or "March" fracture of the second, third or fourth metatarsal bones of the foot. This can occur in healthy individuals through ordinary walking and received the title "March fracture" because it is sustained by relatively untrained soldiers during the course of a fatiguing march. Sometimes the symptoms occur so gradually that the patient cannot believe she has suffered an injury. This means that the fracture may be of several week's duration before advice is sought. There is a "hair-line" crack in the shaft of the bone so fine that x-rays taken during the first few days often fail to disclose it. This factor, together with the delay in reporting the injury, sometimes means that the victim continues her activities, albeit painfully. The continued weight-bearing spreads the inflammatory fracture reaction and causes an excess of callus (the bone-repairing "cement" thrown off by bones after a fracture) to form in the area. Obviously, such a permanent growth is going to be a handicap to such a finely-tuned individual as a dancer.

The victim will complain of pain in the middle of the sole of the foot; sometimes there will be a lump on the top surface of the foot. The treatment is Elastoplast strapping around the foot for three weeks or so; severe cases need a plaster of paris walking plaster. Exercises are given for the toes and weight-bearing restricted during the period of fixation.

When a child fixes her feet at 180° without controlling the hips during early weight-bearing outward rotation exercises, much of that rotational strain is taken on the knees. This can result in permanent misalignment between the foot and the knee, the outward rotation of the hip causing the patella (kneecap) to become dislocated. The patella can also be dislocated through direct violence such as a banging together of knees or knocking against a projection. The kneecap nearly always slides outwards and lies, obviously displaced, on the outside of the knee; there is not much swelling as a rule but there may be severe pain at the time of the injury. Sometimes, the patella goes back into place spontaneously and the diagnosis has to be made on the patient's story of the injury.

This is a serious injury requiring immobilization for anything up to two months; to avoid recurrence, operative treatment is sometimes carried out. Because of the recurrence factor this injury is not a particularly optimistic affair for the dancer. The patella also has a predisposition toward dislocation in a child suffering from a degree of GENU RECURVATUM. This is a condition in which the knees are overextended so that the legs are braced extensively back (See Figs. 21 and 22). This is not an uncommon condition and is often caused by forced stretching of the hamstrings muscles (on the back of the thighs) in children. This is done in an effort to lengthen them and permit greater forward

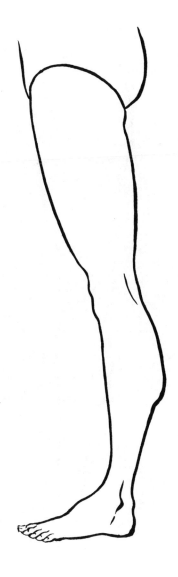

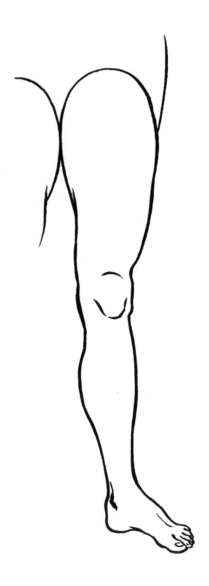

flexion of the body toward the toes. When the hamstrings are tight the ligaments at the back of the knees are stretched and cause the knee to over-brace back.

The shoulder, elbow and jaw are prone to dislocation through the rigors of active exercise, although happily infrequently. A dislocated joint is accompanied by severe and sickening pain, loss of power, considerable swelling and bruising, deformity, and tenderness around the injured joint, which is locked owing to the displacement of the bones involved in the joint. If a dislocation is suspected a doctor should be sent for at once and the teacher should make no attempt to reduce the dislocation, but should steady and support the limb in the position which gives most ease to the patient. If it is necessary to move the injured person, padding can be used to make the journey an easier one by eliminating jolting.

A worrying complication associated with a contusion or severe bruise to a muscle group, such as the thigh muscles, is that with the fearsome name of myositis ossificans traumatica or ossifying hematoma. This takes the form of the gradual collecting or formation of an area of bone-like substance within the actual muscle tissue. For various reasons that are not entirely clear to the medical profession, the capsule of the blood clot which has formed through the hard knock, will harden and eventually become calicified or bone-like, being adherent to the surrounding healthy muscle tissue. Thus a strip of non-elastic "bone" is formed to hinder the smooth action of surrounding healthy elastic muscle fibers.

There is no known predisposition on the part of any one to acquire this condition, nor is it apparently possible to avoid it without being ultra cautious, a safety-first policy hardly in keeping with the normal speed required in treating active injuries. If the teacher notices that a bruised area of muscular tissue is not clearing up satisfactorily with continued normal treatment, that the range of movement of the joint on which the muscle works is becoming progressively less, and that a hard mass can be felt within the muscle itself, then myositis ossificans should be suspected and medical advice sought. One interesting feature of this condition is that an x-ray picture will rarely show the trespassing bone formation until the injury has been in existence for about three weeks.

The treatment consists of the complete cessation of heat and massage, which only serve to aggravate the condition. Rest and gentle nonweight-bearing exercises are carried out, with later rehabilitation consisting mainly of restoring the dancer's sense of balance to compensate for the inelastic substance contained permanently within the muscle, because the "bone" eventually affixes itself to the normal bone of the limb and remains there.

# PART V

# 26

# Back to Work

A "guest" chapter by Lilian Moore *

"Yesterday I went back to class, and I felt wonderful all the way through, but today I can hardly walk." Or: "This will be my first class in three months, and I'm not quite sure what's going to happen!"

How often one hears remarks of this kind in the dressing room of a ballet studio! Very few professional dancers seem to realize that the problem of getting back into practice after an injury, an illness, or merely a pleasant holiday is a matter which requires systematic planning. Energy is no substitute for patience, and uncontrolled enthusiasm can easily lead to disaster.

A dancer can occasionally miss classes for three or four days with no ill effects except a slight insecurity when he returns. After an absence of even so little as one week, however, he should ease into the routine of dancing rather than plunge into it at full strength. This sometimes demands considerable self-control. The results will be worth it, however, for even after a serious and prolonged illness a dancer who has recovered his health should be able to get back into training with no pain or discomfort whatsoever, and—most important of all—with no relapses or setbacks.

---

* (Reprinted, with kind permission of the writer, from "Dancing Times," August, 1964).

If the dancer has simply taken a holiday, the return is merely a matter of setting up a schedule and adhering to it. For example, after being off for one week, he might follow a plan like this:

First day, barre work only; second day, barre and the first exercises in the center; third day, continue all through the exercises in the center, including the adage; fourth day, add the small warm-up jumps and simple pointe work; fifth day, do the entire class.

If such a plan is followed, there should be no stiffness or soreness at all.

An absence of a month would, of course, require an entirely different schedule. Something like this might be indicated: First three days, twenty-minute barre only; next three days, full barre; seventh and eighth days, barre, and center exercises; ninth and tenth days, add the first small jumps; eleventh day, do the entire class.

To the dancer who is young, strong and impatient, this regime may seem too slow and careful. He may feel that he is wasting the first ten days by not doing a complete class. Nevertheless, three weeks after his return from holiday he will in all probability be dancing at top form again, while his colleagues who plunged straight into the most violent exercises will still be struggling with muscle soreness and minor strains, if nothing more disastrous has occurred.

The age of the dancer is, of course, something to be considered. Contrary to popular belief, very young dancers—those not yet twenty—tire more easily and sometimes are more prone to injury than those who have already built up their endurance and are in the age group which, for ballet dancers, seems to have the greatest physical strength: about twenty-two to thirty-two for

women, and twenty-five to thirty-five for men. Since the
youngsters will probably be impatient, it is up to the
teacher to protect them from themselves by not permitting them to work beyond the advisable period.

When a dancer is recovering from an injury or illness, particular care is indicated. He should, of course,
inform the teacher, before he begins the first class, of
the exact nature of the disability he has suffered. He
must also be guided by the advice of his doctor; but unfortunately there are many otherwise highly competent
doctors who do not understand how rigorous and even
gruelling classical ballet exercises can be, and therefore
they sometimes tell dancers that they may start working again before their bodies are ready to undergo the
strain of a full class.

In one instance, a doctor advised a young woman who
was recuperating from hepatitis—a particularly debili-
tating disease—that she could dance "a little, say about
an hour a day." She struggled through a full hour of a
professional class, and became so weak and ill that she
was obliged to rest for another week before trying again.

With the ageing dancer—which may mean someone no
older than thirty—deliberate care in getting back into
practice is of the most vital importance. I know of one
case where a man of about forty, who had been an excellent character dancer, accepted a position as ballet
master and premier of a resident opera company. He
had been physically inactive for about a year (in fact,
he had been engaged in a business enterprise). He spent
only about three weeks getting back into shape, and even
during that time he worked sporadically, for he was
staging and rehearsing the opera ballets and did not de-
vote much attention to his own work. On the opening

night, in the middle of the performance, he wrenched his knee so severely that the muscles and tendons both above and below it were badly torn, and he went straight into hospital. Not only was he unable to fulfill his contract, but he never danced again.

On the other hand, Nicolas Legat, in his charming book, *The Story of the Russian School*, describes how the ballerina Vera Trefilova, with his help, was able to dance again after a ten-year interval:

"Vera Trefilova . . . married and settled down to domestic life, never expected to return to the stage. Long years passed. Then her husband died. She suffered a stroke and fell seriously ill. It appeared that one leg was partially paralyzed. The prospect of dancing again seemed more remote than ever. So I was never so surprised as when one day, after the revolution, she came to me in Petrograd and announced her wish to return to the stage. The problem was a delicate one . . . The first day, despite her impatient tears, I permitted her to work a few minutes only. Next day a little more, and so on. The result was that, without a single complaint of sickness or pain, she regained in three months the technique it had taken years originally to acquire . . ."

After a lengthy interruption for any cause, it is usually best for the professional dancer—unless he is fortunate enough to have a Legat to guide him—to work by himself for some time, before returning to class at all. In working with others there is always a certain amount of tension and strain· The dancer wishes to excel, to please the teacher; if he is unable to execute certain movements properly he is embarrassed by the presence of his colleagues.

In working alone, there is none of this tension. Moreover, the intelligent dancer can plan his exercises so that strength is gradually restored to the weakened part of the body.

With the help and advice of a very wise physician, a young ballerina with a severely torn calf muscle (gastrocnemius) was able to regain full use of it through the following regime:

For six weeks, while the torn tissues were healing, she was permitted no exercise more strenuous than walking. She then started to practice alone; first and second days, ten minutes; third and fourth days, fifteen minutes; of fifth and sixth days, twenty minutes; seventh day, twenty-five minutes (the doctor advised her not to interrupt her practice even on Sundays, while working her way into form). During this week, the calf muscle was further strengthened by an exercise which was done ten times every hour of the day: with the support of a chair back, cabinet or any other convenient article of furniture, the dancer, in stockinged feet, simply rose slowly and carefully to demipointes (in first position) and then lowered the heels in a demi-plié. Although it took only about one minute, this simple exercise, because of the frequency with which it was done, was enormously helpful in restoring the full use of the injured leg.

Second week: first three days, half-hour barre, last four days, 40 minutes, including barre, simple exercises in the center, and traveling turns (deboules and pique turns, to recover the use of the head and the sense of equilibrium in turning, without subjecting the calf muscle to the strain of a quick relevé as in a pirouette).

Third week: first three days, forty-five minutes; next four days, fifty minutes. A few simple jumps (Changements de pied, jetés, etc). were now attempted.

Fourth week: the dancer now worked alone for a full hour every day.

At the beginning of the fifth week she returned to class, although still exercising caution about big, strenuous jumps. Pointe work, with its constant strain on the calf muscle, was not resumed for another fortnight.

At the time, the process of recovery seemed exceedingly slow, and sometimes it was very difficult for the dancer to stick to the arbitrary schedule laid out for her, when she felt quite able to attempt a good deal more. Ten years later, however, she knows that it was worth it. The injured leg recovered its full strength and is a reliable support in thirty-two fouettés or any other test which she may subject it. One of her friends was not so fortunate. She suffered a similar but less severe original injury to the calf muscle, and began to work on it too soon. She has had several recurrences plus other troubles with the same leg (an ankle strain, for example) and is now considered such a bad risk, because of cancelled performance, that managers are very wary about engaging her.

Under ideal conditions, permanent ballet companies might include a gradual "working in" period before the resumption of the full schedule of classes and rehearsals after a summer vacation. However, this is impracticable because no company can be expected to pay rehearsal salary to a dancer who is getting back into shape by working for half an hour a day. Consequently, it is up to the dancer to take the responsibility upon herself, and to make sure that she has planned her resumption of practice so that her body can gradually become accustomed, once more, to the heavy demands she puts upon it. The sympathetic teacher can be enormously helpful, of course, by supplying moral support and understanding, and even by planning and enforcing the necessary regime for the impatient pupil. But it is really the personal obligation of the dancer to be in performance trim when autumn rehearsals commence.

# Appendix I

# Physical Activity During Menstruation

The onset of menstruation affects girls differently. Some have symptoms making them less inclined to do anything active, while others are less affected. All, however, must learn to accept menstruation as a normal physiological process which should not be allowed to interfere with normal activities. Many normal women and girls experience variations in mood throughout the menstrual cycle; these changes may be exaggerated particularly in response to some difficult situation or surroundings. Medical opinion is divided about frequency and the causes of physical changes associated with menstruation. There is a similar lack of agreement about its effect upon physical performance—but there is no question of exercise being harmful to a female even during her menstrual period.

Research indicates that the main effects of menstruation occur about two days before the period actually begins and on the first day of the period before blood-flow is established. This indicates that efficiency is at its lowest level BEFORE and not during menstrual flow. Once flow is fully established, all untoward symptoms vanish. Pre-menstrual discomfort is often associated with low-back pain; this is due to increased relaxation of the pelvic ligaments at this time. Most instances of menstrual backache are due to poor body mechanics—faulty posture, inefficient and incorrect ways of lifting and carrying. During this phase there is often a heavy feeling in the legs, together with constipation. It is claimed that all this can be eased by taking regular exercise. Menstrual discomfort is usually present until flow is fully established; acute spasms of pain may occur prior to this, but they are only momentarily incapacitating. Active exercise accelerates the onset of flow, with swimming as the sole exception, where such a spasm may affect a girl sufficiently to make her stop swimming and sink.

Many eminent doctors and authorities have conducted experiments into this subject; their findings are both interesting and valuable. A sample group of 800 women between the ages of eighteen and forty-five revealed a high incidence of symptoms connected with menstruation; one in nine reported severe pain, irritability and headache; one in sixteen complained of depression and tension and four in five said that their bodies swelled. It has been discovered that women are more accident-prone during the eight days of the premenstruum and menstrual period—50 percent of women admitted to hospital said that their accidents occurred during this period. Other sources claim that there is a loss of physical efficiency, mental drive and stability associated with the eight-day period before and during menstruation. Obviously, this can be expected to have considerable repercussions on the temperamental, highly strung, professional dancer.

What effects can be expected generally that might interfere with the physical proficiency of a dancer's performance or which may upset her psychologically?

There is said to be a slowing of reaction time and efficiency during the pre-menstrual period—as both factors are vital to the perfection of a performance, this could be worrying. But on the other hand, it is known that many female athletes have achieved their best performances during menstruation, when records have been made and Olympic medals won. Generally speaking, most authorities seem to agree that any impairment in athletic performance or loss of efficiency occurs mainly during the pre-menstrual period. Of a control group of 553 physical education students, 59 percent suffered pre-menstrual tension with a corresponding fall off in performance. A further 11 percent who suffered no recognizable symptoms in this phase showed definite fall-off in performance as regards speed, accuracy, strength and fatiguability in both pre-menstrual and menstrual periods.

In considering the position of a female dancer one must assess any possible detrimental effects on her health or her performance through menstrual changes. There are no evidences of any permanent harmful physical effect, although psychological repercussions are possible. Experiments indicate that symptoms during the pre-menstrual and menstrual phases are largely determined by underlying neurotic traits and that they are increased by tension and exciting external situations.

It may well be that in a susceptible girl the strain and competition of performance might increase symptoms to a degree where performance suffered.

For dancers to avoid activity during menstruation is impossible and unnecessary; however, there are a few comments worthy of note. During puberty girls often develop weak abdominal muscles so that too many strong abdominal exercises premenstrually should be avoided.

Pure concentric abdominal work can also cause pain. It was interesting to find that amongst a class of thirty fifteen-year-old girls, prospective ballet dancers, at Royal Ballet School, two were noticeably affected as regards pointwork. I was told that in the interest of these two girls, they would not be passed fit for the professional stage since it was unlikely they would stand up to the extremely hard work and high standards required.

Gymnastics and sport are an essential part of a modern school curriculum; unfortunately increasing academic requirements cause homework to progressively supersede physical activity. In children who are physically developing, this situation has a deleterious effect both on their posture and their general health. Many menstrual problems date from this time.

Enthusiastic pupils may tend to minimize adverse symptoms, believing that absence from classes owing to a constant and regularly occurring disability will diminish their chances of success in a highly competitive field. They avidly believe in the tradition that exercise is a "good thing" for menstrual pain; blindly they cling to the belief inculcated by foolish and unfeeling advisors that the whole thing is psychological and best ignored!

Menstruation is best explained and discussed from a physiological aspect; the psychological factors intrude because of the individual variations in the characters, temperaments, intelligence and personalities of the girls concerned. Real problems can be handled by a Gynecologist; they should not be ignored.

All experienced, mature dancers will have said, "Don't worry, it may never happen," only to mutter wryly, "It always happened!". But it has not prevented them from triumphing over discomfort to give performances of outstanding quality.

## Appendix II

# Fighting Nervousness and Tension

It is NOT unexpected that dancers should suffer from "butterflies in the stomach" before a performance. It would be most unusual if they failed to because circumstances are such that tension is almost inevitable.

Butterflies in the stomach are not peculiar to dancers. Everyone, regardless of her age, interests or activity, runs into this "big moment tension" which hits a person when she is suddenly in a situation where something special is demanded in the way of performance, skill or poise. It is a tension that closes in on a person when a key situation arrives in which she is especially anxious to be at her best—it might be before a big public performance, immediately before having to make a speech or during an interview for a coveted job.

Some persons feel the tension hit them and then it departs as the action starts. Most people find that they remain keyed up and tense, with their hearts beating fast, stomach full of twisting and turning butterflies, muscles tied up and a general feeling of hectic nervousness. This means that their efficiency is impaired and their poise and performance deteriorate. Sometimes the tension is not so apparent in actual symptoms but merely ties them up and makes it impossible for them to move or think with their usual efficiency.

Such tension is the reason why so few people do really well when "the chips are down" or are at their best in moments of great pressure. The causes of it are many and varied and differ with the individual; the only common denominator is that the results are the same for all, inefficient performance, loss of poise and upset of usual form. Some fight it hard, others run away from it by trying to stay away from exciting or important situations. A dancer cannot do the latter, so she must fight it.

The best possible answer is to develop a relaxed personality by a study and application of a simple technique that will pay big dividends next time a big moment comes your way. The best natural sedative—the most effective tension pacifier—is slow, deep, regular breathing. If you can associate with your breathing a conscious "letting-go" of your muscles each time you exhale, so much the better. The moment a dancer feels that tension begins to hit her, she should take a deep breath and then try to keep her breathing slow and deep as long as the situation exists. This will slow things down for her, prevent the tension from building up and help her keep her poise. It is also a good idea, if you know you are approaching a tension situation to begin an emphasis on slow, regular, deep breathing trying to let your muscles go limp and easy on each exhalation. This will often prevent the situation from developing at all.

Try to remember that a few deep breaths, taken slowly and easily, will always help calm you down and set you up for a poised and efficient performance. Quick, shallow breathing is the result of tension and it, in turn, creates more problems. Slow, deep and regular breathing, even when forced, is associated with a feeling of poise and calmness and is the enemy of tension.

# Preventing and Fighting the Common Cold

It is often cold and drafty backstage or in a studio. Waiting around in flimsy costumes renders a dancer prey to the common cold, not in itself a crippling condition but a source of nuisance and highly contagious. Unfortunately, there is still no cure or sure prevention for the common cold, but a great deal can be done to cut down its incidence and severity.

It is an unfortunate thing to say, but there seems to be considerable reason for suggesting that a fit person is more likely to get a cold than an unfit one! The finer condition of the physically fit dancer, which one would assume would be a preventive, appears to be overwhelmed by other factors, associated with physical activity—the loss of Vitamin C through regular and heavy perspiration, for example. If one knows the causes of a condition, then it is easier to take measures to defeat it. By eliminating the factors listed below a great deal can be done to aid the "cold-prone" dancer.

### Causative Factors

1. Not wearing hats outdoors.
2. Sudden changes of body temperature.

3. Loss of Vitamin C through perspiration without sufficient replenishment.

4. Fatigue following hard sessions, often associated with sudden changes of body temperature.

5. Fatiguing activity during the early and mild stages of a cold—also before a cold has properly cleared up.

6. Insufficient protein intake for the work that is being performed.

7. Overconfidence in ability to "shake it off!" Mistaken impression that high standard of physical condition is an iron defence.

8. Chilling during practices.

9. Chilling after a practice of a performance by standing around.

10. Generally inadequate nutrition.

11. Exertion on top of fatigue caused by lack of sleep or insufficient recovery from previous effort.

12. Careless attitude regarding proper drying of head before going out in cold; wearing insufficient clothing, etc.

An "anti-cold" campaign could be put into operation when the severe weather begins, with emphasis on the fact that all precautions taken are part of the training procedure of the dancer and that each dancer has an obligation to observe them. It is also a demonstrable fact that results improve when a person is told the reason for each suggested procedure. For example—

ALWAYS WEAR A HAT WHEN THE WEATHER TURNS BRISK. Why? In order to protect the body from sudden temperature changes following exertion when resistance is lower than usual. Explain that temperature change lowers bodily resistance and the subject should—during activity, afterwards and in her general life—try to sustain regular body temperature, avoiding chilling situations.

AVOID STANDING AROUND DURING AND AFTER PRACTICE IN COLD WEATHER. Plan practice so that everyone is always on the move. If this is not possible see that the people not in action are adequately clothed and protected from the weather. Instruct everyone not to stand around out of doors after practices are concluded. Get work going quickly before dancers get cold.

EAT PLENTY OF VITAMIN C FOODS AND SUPPLEMENT IF NECESSARY. Explain that Vitamin C is an anti-infective vitamin and helps combat secondary infections associated with colds. In winter, the consumption of citrus fruits drops and the regular intake of Vitamin C is cut down. Since this vitamin is not stored, but must constantly be replenished, foods containing it must be given a top priority. Also explain that Vitamin C is lost in perspiration, thus a greater need for it is created. Suggest a dancer eats as many oranges as possible each day and at least a glass of tomato juice per day. Vitamin C can also be taken in tablet form—three 100 milligram tablets, one per meal. If a person has any sign of a cold or has just been exposed to chilling and/or fatigue, give six of these tablets per day for two or three days. This control has demonstrated excellent results, especially in lessening the severity of colds and preventing secondary infections.

USE ADEQUATE RECOVERY TECHNIQUES AFTER HARD PRACTICES. To avoid infections developing when a dancer is fatigued, be sure that there is a proper cooling off period after activity. Also, use a graduated training and conditioning program to avoid excessive fatigue. When a person is excessively fatigued be sure she avoids chilling and has a good post-effort meal and a chance to rest.

BE CAUTIOUS ABOUT LETTING PEOPLE WITH MILD COLD SYMPTOMS OR WHO ARE RECOVERING FROM A COLD, WORK VERY HARD. Of course, this is a rule that is extremely difficult to apply in any walk of life and particularly in the dancing world! Everyone should be taught to take notice of any signs of colds, and should not undertake heavy work at this time. If a dancer does work or practice during this period, she should be sure to take full anti-chilling precautions afterwards regardless of how good she may feel.

REST, VITAMIN C AND PROTEIN AT THE FIRST SIGNS OF INFECTION. If a person shows possible cold symptoms suggest the liberal use of oranges and tomato juice, as much rest as possible and plenty of protein food. Explain how such a procedure, especially rest, in the first hour of a cold can often cut it dead or at least lessen its severity. If a person has any suspicions of a cold coming, she should not be optimistic—take all precautions anyway. People who work hard but have low protein food percentage in their diet are more prone to colds, especially heavy colds and other more serious infections. Hard working male dancers should get at least 125, but preferably 150-200 gms. of protein per day. There are two types of protein—animal and vegetable protein. The former consists of cheese, corned beef, mutton and eggs primarily; the latter can be peanuts, wholemeal flour, peas, spinach, potatoes, carrots, turnips.

EXPLAIN THAT GOOD PHYSICAL CONDITION IS NOT A SURE ARMOUR. Be sure that the dancers understand that they are more sensitive to infection when they are in a high state of physical fitness. This is due to body temperature changes, perspiration, fatigue, etc. They should be taught to act accordingly and that it is intelligent and not "soft" to take sensible precautions. They should not let "kidding" by unfit friends force them into casual behavior.

THE ROLE OF SLEEP. Lack of sleep lowers resistance, so that extra precautions are needed when people are tired. The importance of sleep after hard effort must be stressed. Lack of sleep when cold symptoms are present will greatly increase chances of the cold developing into a serious one, possibly a major infection.

PRECAUTIONS AND EXPOSURE. People should avoid contacts with people having colds as much as possible. Whenever exposed in this way, take precautions by getting extra rest, avoiding excessive fatigue and increasing Vitamin C and protein intake. Kissing people who have colds is a very easy, if pleasant, method of receiving infection!

It is only by constantly repeating these facts that a "cold-consciousness" will be developed. Probably the greatest single factor, and the one most easily put into practice, is that of fighting colds by means of nutrition. A proper diet provides the best possible armour against infections, a good Vitamin C and protein intake must be sustained and a dancer MUST replenish her body thorougly after hard effort.

Some of the tougher characters among us like to try and "sweat out" a cold by intense activity. If the cold is a mild one and there is no temperature or indication of sore throat, swollen glands or severe headache, then a good physical workout often seems to help in getting rid of a cold. However, the work should not be so severe that it exhausts the subject; she needs as much energy as possible to fight off any possible infection. When in any doubt, consult a doctor but most houses have a thermometer handy and if there is any temperature present then don't take a chance!

If a person has had what is termed a "common cold" she can return to work as soon as it departs, providing she has not had a high temperature, in which case it is wise to wait at least twenty-four hours after the temperature has gone down. If it has been a cold of the influenza type, it is wise to be very careful about when a person returns to full duty. Flu often leaves one in a weakened condition, and it is suggested that the doctor give permission before she returns to work.

A readily available aid in fighting off colds and other infections, besides giving a general feeling of well-being to a person, is the regular use throughout the winter months of an artificial sunlight lamp. Nowadays there is no need for anyone to suffer from the effects of lack of sunshine because synthetic sunshine can be obtained from ultra-violet light lamps. The most important quality of sunlight is not the healthy looking tan it gives—there is more to it than that. It improves the general health, increases the appetite and has a beneficial effect upon muscular performance. Repeated small doses of ultra-violet light increase the capacity for work and the efficiency with which it is carried out; under its action the oxygen used by the body for any given piece of work is reduced.

Ultra-violet rays increase the blood supply in the skin, the pigmentation which follows increases the resistance of the skin while the shorter rays destroy organisms on the skin's surface and fight off acne, boils and other common skin complaints. The irradiation of the skin causes changes in the blood which increase the resistance of the body to infection such as colds and bronchitis.

# Index